RITUALS OF CARE

RITUALS OF CARE

Karmic Politics in an Aging Thailand

Felicity Aulino

CORNELL UNIVERSITY PRESS   ITHACA AND LONDON

First published 2019 by Cornell University Press

Library of Congress Cataloging-in-Publication Data

Names: Aulino, Felicity, author.
Title: Rituals of care : karmic politics in an aging Thailand / Felicity Aulino.
Description: Ithaca : Cornell University Press, 2019. | Includes bibliographical
   references and index.
Identifiers: LCCN 2019009363 (print) | LCCN 2019011862 (ebook) |
   ISBN 9781501739743 (pdf) | ISBN 9781501739750 (epub/mobi) |
   ISBN 9781501739729 | ISBN 9781501739729 (cloth) |
   ISBN 9781501739736 (pbk.)
Subjects: LCSH: Older people—Care—Thailand—Chiang Mai. | Caregivers—
   Thailand—Chiang Mai. | Older people—Thailand—Chiang Mai—Social
   conditions. | Buddhism—Social aspects—Thailand—Chiang Mai. | Population
   aging—Social aspects—Thailand—Chiang Mai. | Ethnology—Thailand—
   Chiang Mai.
Classification: LCC HV1484.T55 (ebook) | LCC HV1484.T55 A95 2019 (print) |
   DDC 362.609593—dc23
LC record available at https://lccn.loc.gov/2019009363

To my parents

Contents

Acknowledgments

So many wonderful people made this project possible and have supported me through the years of research and writing. I am told the acknowledgments cannot be longer than the book itself, so here I will name but a few of the generous souls who have made this experience so very rich. To the friends, the funders, and the winds of fate that helped bring this work to fruition—I thank you so.

Deepest thanks go to my friend and mentor Linchong Pothiban, of Chiang Mai University's Faculty of Nursing. She set this project on its course and nurtured me and my family every step of the way. Immense gratitude also goes to Sawang Kaewkantha, who was a constant guide and ally, and who opened up the world of elder care in Thailand to me.

I use pseudonyms for most of the people who appear in this book, though I am deeply grateful for their every assistance, great and small. Words in fact cannot express the gratitude I feel for everyone who allowed me to occupy the strange role of anthropologist and to live and work in their midst. Particular thanks goes to my family in Nong Hoi.

The research and writing represented here was made possible by generous grant support. My thanks go to the Social Science Research Council, the Wenner-Gren Foundation, the Harvard Committee on General Scholarships, the Mellon Foundation, and the Templeton Foundation.

Thanks unending to Mary-Jo DelVecchio Good, my mentor since college, without whom none of this would have been possible; Byron Good, an intellectual interlocutor beyond compare; Arthur Kleinman, an incredibly generous teacher, reader, and guide; Michael Herzfeld, an ally with great taste and superb attention to detail; and Michael Puett, whose enthusiasm and insight have proven inspirational at every turn. Michael M. J. Fischer has shown me what masterful scholarship looks like, and I thank him for his feedback on this project. Charles Hallisey remains a steadfast guide. Thank you to Paul Farmer, Anne Becker, Salmaan Keshavjee, and Arthur Kleinman, and the entire crew of Societies of the World 25, who taught me an enormous amount about global health practice and pedagogy, greatly influencing my thinking. Thank you to all my teachers, including the late Stanley J. Tambiah, who was a good friend and through whom I came to appreciate the power of history and the disorienting strength of radical egalitarianism. And above all, thank you to Aba Cecile McHardy, the Friendly Dragon, a guide in life and scholarship to whom I remain devoted across lifetimes; her influence can be marked on every page.

In Thailand, countless friends have guided my way and my understanding. A particularly warm thanks goes to Tana Nilchaikovit, from whom I have learned so much on so many levels. Deep appreciation, too, to Komatra Chuengsatiansup, a great mentor at home and abroad. Thank you to those working tirelessly with and for older people: Ajarn Aphassree Cheikuna, Phannaphat Mam Phophaenna, Janevit Wisojsongkram, Saranyu Win Kaewkantha, P'A, P'Jeu, Sirinat Sonia Kasikam, Nong X, Sirinapa O-way, Nong Eunjai, Usa Khierwrord, and Somporn Nok Kiokaew. Additional thanks to Nong Way for her assistance, along with Sukyunya Pornsopakul, Duen Heang, and the incomparable Sangwan Poo Palee. Thanks go to the palliative care experts who taught me so much, including Veeramonl Chantaradee, Dr. Issarang Nuchprayoon, Wasinee Wisesrith, and Dr. Mano Laohavanich. Special thanks to the palliative care team at the Songklanagarind Hospital, Prince Songkla University, in Hat Yai, including Temsak Phungrassami, Sakon Singha, P'Fong, and P'Yae. Thanks also to everyone at the Phuthikā Network, including Phra Paisal Wisalo and Sui Wanna Jarusombun. Thanks to Win Pop Mektri and to everyone at the Volunteer Spirit Network for generous access to the library. And my gratitude to the incredible scholars, policymakers, and practitioners for their time, work, and generosity, including John Knodel, Wipada Kunaviktikul, Wichit Sisopan, Siriphan Sasat, Bprasaan Tangchai, Tanet Wongyanawa, Naret Songkrawsook, Khwanchai Visithanon, Virapun Wirojratana, Samrit Srithamrongsawat, Suriya Wongkongkrathep, Weerasak Muangpaisan, P'Kaek, and Usamard Siampukdee.

A lifetime of gratitude to all my amazing colleagues in the Pioneer Valley for their support and inspiration in growing this work, including (but not at all limited to) Sonya Atalay, Elif Babül, Whitney Battle-Baptiste, Sue Darlington, Chris Dole, Deborah Gewertz, Alan Goodman, Suzanne Gottschang, Jennifer Hamilton, Krista Harper, Maria Heim (a game changer), Julie Hemment, Betsy Krause, Tom Leatherman, Lynne Morgan, Joshua Roth, Andy Rotman, Sahar Sadjadi, Boone Shear, Pam Stone, and Jackie Urla. Thank you to the Five Colleges and everyone in Culture, Health, and Science. And thank you Jen Sandler for critical relationality, and for guiding me to others naming and practicing transformative change.

My gratitude to Tanya Luhrmann for including me in the Mind and Spirit Project, which gave final direction to this work, and to the crew: Josh Brahinsky, John Dulin, Emily Ng, Rachel Smith, plus Kara Weisman, Vivian Dzokoto, and Nikki Ross-Zehnder. Hard to single out, but, Josh, thank you for the structuring commutes; and Emily, thank you for reading and naming and g-chatting through it all.

Thank you and continued loyalty to the original Thai writing group: Eli Elinoff, Malavika Reddy, Claudio Sopranzetti, and Benjamin Tausig. Claudio, you made it all possible—as friend and brother, we delight in and count on knowing you in the world. Lisa Stevenson, thank you for everything, for getting and supporting it all. And heartfelt thanks to other colleagues, friends, teachers, and family (and all combinations thereof) for their immense instrumental support, great insight, and good humor: Adisorn Juntrasook, Addy and Nick Grossman, Adia Benton, Akiko Mori, Andrew Johnson, Anna Corwin, Aroon Puritat, Barbara Barry, Bob Bickner, all the wonderful Thai teachers and my fellow students in Madison, Bonnie Brereton, Brooke Schedneck, Carey Clouse, Charlie Carstens, Chuck and Molly, Diarra Lamar, Donald Swearer, Eduardo Kohn, Elana Buch, Emiko Ohnuki, Erick White, everyone at the land foundation, Gernot Huber, Jamie Burford, Jason Danely, Jeffrey Samuels, Jeremy Smith, Jo Cook, Joe Harris, Julia Cassaniti, Kristina Lyons, Kurt Wise, Larry Ashmun, Kate Mason, Margaret Wiener, Marilyn Goodrich, Marisa Guptarak, Matt Yoxall, Mau Daw, Milena Marchesi, Mook MS, Mui Cheewintha Boon-Long, Nick Thomson, Non Arkaraprasertkul, Oriana Walker, Peggy Aulino, Pote Videt, Rachel Broudy, Raeann LeBlanc, Rebecca Hall, Roseanne Carrara, Saipin Suputtamongkol, Scott Stonington (a gem in the world, partner in this work), Shika Card, Smita Lahiri, Toby Lee, Tom Blair, Tom Borchart, Vicky Koski-Karell, Wirun Limsawart, Yoko Hayami, and Yuyang Mei. I could write pages on each and every one of you; such warmth to you all! Anitra Grisales, thank you for taking me on and providing insight and a formidably edited path to follow. And thanks, too, to Jim Lance, peer reviewers, and everyone at Cornell University Press for supporting this book—thrilling beyond belief.

I learned a lot about caregiving—its mixtures of sacrifice and devotion and love and simply showing up—perhaps most vividly in my own home. My mom spent eleven hours a day with us, caring for baby Ren her first year as I wrote the first iteration of this book, and my dad endured so much time alone to let her go. In the years since, they have done all the more, from the daily for baby Eamonn to reading these words and cheering me on. And sweetest Kevin Moore, a second dedication to you and the kiddos too for making this with me, wondrously turning all trials and travails into adventures. I love you.

Note on Names and Thai Transliteration

Names have been changed to protect the privacy of the people in this book, except for public figures speaking on the record.

Throughout, I use primarily the Romanization scheme of the American Library Association—Library of Congress (ALA-LC) for transliteration of the Thai language. Exceptions include abbreviations and words commonly transliterated otherwise (such as *jai* for ใจ, as opposed to the formal ALA-LC *čhai*).

RITUALS OF CARE

AN INVITATION TO CARE

Boonyuang takes hold of her mother by the armpits and yanks her up to the top of her bed with several rapid, forceful movements. A slight grimace passes over the older woman's face and is quickly gone. It is the first changing of the day, and, softly muttering "dirty, dirty" (*sokaprok, sokaprok*, สกปรก ๆ), Boonyuang gets on with her routine. She tosses aside the top sheet and unfastens her mother's nighttime diaper. The pungent smell of loose stool fills their small room, as Boonyuang pushes her mother's semi-paralyzed frame over onto her left hip to gain access to her backside. With gruff and practiced hands, she makes quick work of cleaning and powdering. As she affixes a new diaper with a twisting configuration of rubber bands, she explains that the sticky tape provided on the Pampers' ends is not strong enough to hold the sides together. Months of trial and error have led to the system now in place. Boonyuang next reaches for a scrub brush and lifts her mother's one usable hand up as she whisks back and forth across dainty nails soiled by self-exploration. Each action is rough and unapologetic, and at the same time skilled and effective. Boonyuang deftly moves the elder's legs into a pair of brightly patterned pants to finish the job, and deposits the bedding into a basin for her next task of the day.

Boonyuang, at age seventy, is the primary caregiver for her bedridden ninety-two-year-old mother, Yāi Maw.[1] The two live together in Chiang Mai's old town, the inner moated area of the largest city in Northern Thailand. Situated behind a modest faux-brick house off a narrow alleyway that snakes behind the white exterior wall of an ornate temple close to the northern wall of the city, their wooden home is reminiscent of a traditional Lanna-style dwelling—though instead of an

1

open-air ground floor, the lower portion of the structure has been enclosed. Boonyuang rents out the upper level, leaving only the cramped underside, with wooden plank walls and ceilings no more than five feet high, for her and her mother. Boonyuang is not much more than four feet tall, and her mother cannot sit up, so they somehow manage (without having to duck, unlike some visitors) as they go about their daily affairs.

Yāi Maw had been a vegetable seller for decades. She used to carry regularly two heavy baskets balanced on her shoulder with a long pole, work that led to her increasing discomfort over the years. She is now largely deaf, nearly blind, and entirely incontinent, with excruciating pain in her back and no desire (or ability) to leave the house. She spends her days and nights on a donated hospital bed, its metal arms raised to keep her penned in, with a partial view to the outside world through the slatted panes of a small window and the screen of the door, when open. On her bed just within reach lie a blue plastic flashlight and a back scratcher. The metal table beside her is lined with pill bottles, packages of crackers, and a cup with a bendy straw, along with a transistor radio, which is either turned up to full volume or droning quietly, unnoticed. Behind her, above the head of Boonyuang's bed, which takes up the remainder of their one room, an array of pictures covers the wall: several revered monks; the nation's king; a bright eight-by-twelve portrait of an older man, Boonyuang's late husband, set against a background of bright blue sky and white puffy clouds; a photograph of a beautiful young woman, Boonyuang's daughter, clad in a university uniform, complete with white collared shirt and half smile. These are deceased family members, departed too soon.[2]

Boonyuang will shortly perch on a stool outside, bent over three buckets. She gets going with the wash in a small orange bucket, the type sold around town filled with toiletries and other necessities to be donated to Buddhist monks clad in robes of the same hue. Once scrubbed, the sheets are transferred to another soap-filled bucket, this one pink. Boonyuang puts her back into the motions as she stoops, lifts, and repeats, concluding with a final rinse with plain water in the largest of the plastic vessels. After the balance of water is wrung out, the laundry is hung to dry, looking like oversized prayer flags on lines crisscrossing the side yard. On my first visit, Boonyuang remarks as she washes that she does this three or four times per day. Occasionally a volunteer from a local nongovernmental organization (NGO) will stop by with some offering of money, brochures, or community news; some days a visitor turns up with sweets or a fresh supply of diapers. And so my introduction to care in this northern city of Thailand begins.

The scene can be astonishing at first pass. An aged daughter and her elderly mother in an impossibly small room, stuffed with first-aid supplies, with an endless stream of chores to keep their humble household running. But it has been this way for years. However unsettling the state of affairs may seem to outsiders witnessing it for the first time, the situation has become ordinary. And it is this very ordinariness that I seek to explore in this book. My focus is care in the everyday, and the ordinary is the route by which I want to bring attention to the habituated ways people provide for one another—not only at bedsides, but also in boardrooms, corner stores, or any number of mundane daily interactions. This focus illustrates that care is not universally parsed as a matter of concern and assistance, but rather is a function of the ways people's attention is trained by the social world to perceive and prioritize what needs to be done, and for whom, and in what ways.

The ethnographic scenes depicted in this book will appear both familiar and strange to many readers. Thailand, this relatively small nation of sixty-six million people in mainland Southeast Asia, faces struggles similar to many other places in the world, including a rapidly aging population, the exploitation of the working and middle classes, and economic and authoritarian roadblocks to political participation. People care for the sick and provide for their communities amid such conditions, and much of what they do can be described, using familiar analytic concepts, as reflecting and resisting a variety of social pressures. But Thailand is also predominantly Buddhist, one of many indications of the powerful influence of centuries-old practice and philosophical lineages, distinct from European traditions, evident in arenas large and small, personal and political. Getting a handle on the sensibilities instilled by this social world is what I seek here. Close attention to mundane affairs—from home-care routines to friendly social interactions, from volunteer home visits to professional conference presentations—invites an appreciation of the subtle logics of engagement from which lived experience here stems.

Take a classic volunteer visit as a simple example. Yāi Maw's neighborhood volunteer arrived one day around New Year with a caravan from a nearby older people's organization. The team disembarked from the NGO's tall, white, ten-passenger vehicle and wound their way back to the entrance of Boonyuang's house, all in matching collared polo shirts and neatly pressed slacks. They held a brightly colored silk scarf folded tidily and encased in clear plastic. Greetings were exchanged as the group gracefully arranged themselves around the bed, squeezing in without disturbing any of the pair's belongings, despite the tight space. The mood was markedly jovial, and everyone showered Yāi Maw with compliments on her strength and the skill of Boonyuang's caretaking. They then presented the scarf as a gift, helping to arrange the old woman's hands to accept the package. Everyone found some way to place a hand on the receiver as the offering was bestowed, whether directly or indirectly by touching the elbow of someone else closer in, forming a chain of merit made and captured by dozens of camera flashes. And as quickly as they had come, they were merrily off to their next destination.

In the chapters of this book, I hope to provide a sense of how and why situations like this are calibrated care in context. The perfunctoriness of the visit above in some ways mimics typical trips to Thai Buddhist temples, as I explore in chapter 1 in terms of the karma of care. The preparation of the items offered is essential, and neatness of presentation is well tended. The actions count and must be executed according to guiding parameters. When followed, there is social and spiritual care enacted in these forms, from the alleviation of karmic burdens to a resultant sense of comfort. That no one directly probed into the emotional well-being of Yāi Maw and Boonyuang is also fairly typical, as I discuss in chapter 2 in terms of the conditioning of care, representing a logic of psychosocial support geared to draw people's focus away from their troubles and distress. The formality of the visit, even the height of people's hands raised in greeting, indicates to all the relative status of members of the group. As people maneuver their bodies following the dictates of polite hierarchy, the nearly scripted sets of movements provide a felt stability to the gathering, even if temporarily. Such deployments of perception and power are discussed in chapter 3 in terms of care of the social body, and in chapter 5 in regard to the violence of care.

One might be tempted to focus on the abundance of resources expended in the affair sketched above; the event might then seem hollow, not only for the token offering but for the fleeting time spent "volunteering" in such an encounter. In turn, the scene could be enlisted to challenge a host of community aid projects that spend a great deal of time in a similar fashion. But while at some level such critique is warranted, as explored in the civic landscape of care presented in chapter 4, this scene can also reveal aspects of how people do meaningfully provide for one another, even if and when also failing to alleviate pressing burdens or enabling oppressive power relations. Attention to appearance, the correct application of ritual-type technologies, and hierarchical deference serve to decenter dominant Euro-American notions of functional utility, disrupt presumptions regarding the importance of sincerity and other psychological components of good care, and reflect important forms of care, however antithetical to egalitarian sensibilities such forms may be.

Indeed, in this book I aim to show how a focus on care can challenge and refine core anthropological concepts. Throughout, I trace how people's attention is trained in Northern Thailand to enable the embodying of appropriate forms, and how little emphasis is placed on cultivating an authentic desire to provide for others. This changes the moral calculus of care as it is commonly conceived and helps draw out the particularities of underlying conceptions of the self. In turn, the stakes and the potential of "care" come into new focus.

I also find a focus on care offers a fresh angle on recent turmoil in Thailand from the vantage point—unusual for political analyses—of embodied practice. Ultimately, given the present struggle over existing norms in Thailand, I argue that the modes of being that are described here, through attention to everyday occurrences in Thai settings, can help open avenues for prompting radical change in settings worldwide, at both individual and structural levels. This is inspired not via abstract and universalizing calls to "care," but through appreciation and transformation of mundane, habituated practices of providing for others.

Originations: From Dying to Aging to Living in the Everyday

I first met Boonyuang and Yāi Maw, along with a host of others discussed in this book, by way of a volunteer-based home-care project for elders in the Chiang Mai municipal area. In 2008, I partnered with this group—what I will call the Older People's Organization, or OPO—as a home base from which to study end-of-life care and the budding hospice movement in Thailand. A strategic alliance among prominent medical doctors, health-care personnel, and "Engaged Buddhist" activists had placed end-of-life at the center of overarching social change efforts in the country. Hospice and palliative care services offer an alternative to biomedicine's typical focus on cure—offering instead attention to physical, mental, and spiritual well-being. In a country in which an estimated 90–95 percent of the population is Buddhist, religious teachings can provide powerful rhetoric within the biomedical establishment as well as compelling practices in the personal realm. These end-of-life advocates in turn were harnessing Buddhist frameworks to change not only the culture of hospital death and home and community care for the dying, but also forms of interpersonal engagement in nearly every sector. I thus sought to explore what constitutes end-of-life care in different contexts, as well as how care for the dying had become a vehicle for large-scale social action.

OPO offered me entree to the homes of families caring for bedridden elders who, one might suspect, were prime candidates for this end-of-life movement. But as I began to work with these elder people and their caregivers, I realized that they did not talk about death in the ways I had been primed to expect by the palliative care literature. In clinical settings around the world, an inability to accept imminent death can lead to heroic lifesaving techniques that are not only costly, but often also increase the suffering of the patient and their loved ones. Terms such as "end of life" (*rayasutthāi khǭng chīwit*, ระยะสุดท้ายของชีวิต, literally "last stage of life") are therefore essential for hospice, as they signal when a person is in need of a different orientation to care. But the people I met through OPO rarely used or volunteered terms like "end of life," or even the more colloquial "close to death" (*klai tāi*, ใกล้ตาย). They were not focused on cure, and resistance to end-of-life language seemed more than simply a fear of or inability to "confront death peacefully," as core trainings of Thai palliative care promote. People were caring in a different register.

A core strength of the ethnographic method is the ability to recognize when one's research focus is projecting significance onto one area when what matters more to people lies elsewhere. I was faced with people caring in a different and seemingly important register, and it gradually dawned on me that my original research questions regarding "care for the dying" had an undue biomedical bias. The term "end of life," so essential to hospice and palliative care discourse, is a relatively new, medically inflected phrase. It indexes a clinically rendered terminal prognosis, which is required to determine whether a person is in the so-called last stages of life and thus qualifies for hospice. Once a person qualifies, a range of services can be enacted to help prompt a "peaceful death" for all involved. Not only did home caregivers not use words like "end of life" and "peaceful death," the long-term care routines they performed every day spoke to a way of being that was unrecognized by this rhetoric. Long-term care routines necessitated bodily action over and above the prognostic recognition and contemplation emphasized by hospice advocates. These routines manifested a mix of practicality, belief, and tradition in the everyday. A research focus on dying seemed an imposition on ordinary experience, experience that was itself worth exploring.

I therefore altered my research so as not to have my questions narrowly defined by the medical gaze, starting instead with the experience of lay caregivers for dependent elders and the organizations that support such work. I then came to appreciate the palliative care movement as it was cast in relief by a set of national platforms on aging and eldercare. Like their hospice counterparts, Thai "population aging" initiatives traded in international best practices, were steeped in Buddhist rhetoric, and aspired to spark social change in relation to a host of attitudes and practices.[3] But unlike the bulk of palliative care efforts, eldercare initiatives were able to escape the centripetal force of biomedicine—at least in some ways.[4] In turn, those providing eldercare ultimately reoriented my understanding of care more generally.

With the focus on eldercare came another proximate backdrop for analysis: population aging. Epidemiological and demographic transitions, economic forces, and new medical technologies have coalesced to increase long-term care needs in many societies. In turn, a political discourse of crisis is emerging around the world, as governments fashion trade agreements that include provisions for the movement of care workers and domestic programs attempt to meet the shifting care demands of citizens. "Aging preparedness" is a guiding buzzword. And, amid grand visions of restoring elders' rightful place as esteemed members of society, the burden of physical care everywhere continues to fall largely on families, women, and marginalized peoples.

Thailand provides a prime example of this overall trend of population aging. Two generations of family planning efforts (beginning in the 1960s) reduced the total fertility rate from six children per woman to fewer than two, while medical advances increased life expectancy by about a decade during the same period. "Older people" (defined as those over the age of sixty) now make up over 13 percent of the total population, a percentage expected to increase steadily in the coming decades.[5] These older people are said to face the prospect of dependency without traditional safety nets, as young people work outside the home to support their families and no longer have a large sibling base with whom to share the responsibilities of providing both monetarily and physically for their elders. Issues of eldercare are prominent in Thai society, as demographers and global health organizations trumpet the country's "aging society" status, and personal narratives and national policies alike draw on a host of models circulating globally to address population inversions.[6]

Anthropologists have grappled in recent years with transformations of social norms caused by growing elder populations. Whether in terms of emergent "elderscapes" (Danely 2015) and "cultural scripts" (Long 2005), thwarted expectations and dominating "decline narratives" (Gullette 2004), or growing pressures to "reimagine" possibilities for eldercare, people around the world seem to be struggling with what will happen to them and to their societies as they age.[7] Indeed, the changes signaled by new idealized visions for old age and long-term care are not superficial. They entail corresponding changes in religious ideology and cultural logics, as well as economic circumstances and social welfare systems (Lamb 2009). And although anthropologists are keen to point out false claims of universality in transnational discourse, such as found in the "successful aging" movement, recognizing the values, cultural assumptions, and political motivations built into circulating models of aging and long-term care, as important as that work is, may not be enough.[8] Changes predicted and heralded by international demographic discourse must not dominate anthropological analysis of population aging, leaving room instead to appreciate subtle (and not-so-subtle) ruptures, continuities, and new formations in people's lives. In turn, insights from eldercare can be shown to have great relevance for a broad range of social analyses.

The set of circumstances surrounding aging and eldercare in Thailand warrants consideration not only by those interested in health and caregiving issues, but also by those engaged in social and political struggles the world over. OPO, as I will describe, is one of the many programs springing up around the country with the explicit purpose of bracing for anticipated age-related social change in Thailand.[9] Like their counterparts in the hospice movement, these programs start from a seemingly narrow set of goals (related to the well-being of older people) and quickly move out to a series of aspirations for societal relations more generally. Both eldercare and hospice advocates in Thailand aspire to ideal visions for open communication and health equity that require massive adjustments to the status quo. Yet their orientation to and promotion of such radical ideals, somewhat counterintuitively, remain enmeshed with traditional logics of care. And while both "movements" largely shied away from the more prominent and politically charged social change efforts bubbling up, and in fact boiling over, at the time of my research, I came to find that their work was bound up with issues underlying the increasingly contentious political landscape, too.

The bulk of my fieldwork for this project took place over sixteen months in 2008 and 2009. Street protests were omnipresent. The dominance and import of political battles during this time forced questions regarding social organization, political legitimacy, and the nature of widespread social change into this study as another necessary backdrop. One corner of Chiang Mai was cordoned off for months, home to a day-in-and-day-out Red Shirt demonstration composed in large part of supporters of the recently ousted and still wildly popular Prime Minister Thaksin Shinawatra. In November 2008, Yellow Shirts—composed mainly of royalists and their sympathizers opposed to Thaksin—managed to close the Suvarnabhumi Airport in Bangkok for eight days of demonstrations, in an attempt to shut down the government and garner international attention to their fight against Thaksin's influence in national affairs. "Reds" barricaded the ASEAN summit in the south in April in a similar move to draw international attention to undemocratic manipulation of the political process. Later that month, the leader of the "Yellows" survived an assassination attempt. Fueled by protests across the country, tensions rose to a fever pitch, culminating in a deadly military crackdown on Red protesters in the commercial center of Bangkok in 2010. And that was only one round of the contemporary crisis, which in many ways began with protests against Thaksin in 2005 and evolved through a series of color-coded reorganizations and city shutdowns that ultimately led to a military takeover of the country in 2014.[10]

The dizzying back and forth of the last decade or so of Thai politics, discussed in broader historical and geopolitical context below, affected lobbying for eldercare initiatives as well as interpersonal dynamics within civil society organizations and the communities they served. But more profoundly, and perhaps more unexpectedly, these larger political contests, I discovered, were interconnected with the embodied routines at the very heart of home caregiving as well. Trying to understand the lived experience of care as practiced at bedsides forced me to consider care as practiced in more general ways—from care for one's group to care for the nation as a whole. What I found was a set of logics that manifested physically as well as ideologically, distinct sensibilities that guided practice in personal and political realms alike. And thus, as I worked to unravel the knot of influences playing out within any given household or any particular aid project, I came to place caregiving in context and to understand Thai politics in a new way.

I came to see that religious, social, and political structures are embodied (and continually resubstantiated) in habituated practices of providing for others. "Caring," rather than being a universal orientation, comprises culturally contingent sets of emotional and practical ways of being with people. An examination of these practices reveals specific historical lineages to each, proving an inseparable link between forms of social organization and forms of care. In turn, ordinary care, in practice, turns out to be a powerful tool for assessing not only enduring modes of moral experience, but also pivotal elements of social change. Rather than the generally flat rendering of lived experience reflected in grand pronouncements of demographic change or political revolution, the everyday stakes and requisite malleability of such large-scale shifts come into focus through detailed attention to ordinary acts of care.

Structures of Adjustment, Infrastructures of Care

Without question, much has changed in the social, political, and economic landscape of Thailand in recent decades. Between 1986 and 1996, Thailand had the fastest-growing GDP in the world, accompanied by major increases in life expectancy, literacy, commodities, and services.[11] Thailand did not follow the Washington Consensus in achieving such growth (a set of prescribed, market-based policy reforms for development), taking instead a strong state approach like that of the so-called Asian Tiger economies, at least at first.[12] But after 1993, it liberalized its market in an attempt to further increase growth, leading to a flood of foreign capital and a boom in real estate speculation. The subsequent bubble burst, in 1997, in what is known as the Asian financial crisis, caused by speculative attacks, the withdrawal of massive amounts of capital, and the free fall of the Thai baht. This shock to the system led to the Thai government's acceptance of an International Monetary Fund recovery program (following a pattern made legible by Naomi Klein 2007; see also Kasian 2015); but the structural adjustments demanded by these IMF loans led to a greater free fall of the economy and a major popular backlash against such policies. As I will show, these changes are profoundly relevant to the provision of care, both institutionally and individually.

This was the backdrop to the 2001 victory of the Thai Rak Thai Party (TRT) and the election of Thaksin Shinawatra as prime minister. At that moment, Thaksin united a diverse set of camps—from venture capitalists to anticapitalists, from royal liberals to avid Marxists—with promises that read to all as casting off the neoliberal yoke of structural adjustment. Running on an unprecedentedly clear policy platform of "Think New, Act New, for All Thais," Thaksin presented a mixture of social welfare and pro-trade inventiveness that came to be known as "Thaksinomics."[13] He immediately set to implementing a series of populist programs, including a village debt moratorium, inexpensive loan strategies, government-guided local business ventures, and the "30-Baht Scheme" for universal health-care coverage.[14] His policies were enormously popular, with fulfilled campaign promises that for once took seriously the rural and urban poor as real constituencies. But as his popularity with the majority of the country increased, a mounting opposition also grew. Among opponents' many complaints were the extrajudicial killings and human rights abuses in Thaksin's draconian war on drugs, widespread corruption, the state-fueled escalation of tensions between Muslims and Buddhists in Thailand's deep south, a broad offensive against the organizing capacity of NGOs and civil society activists, and what were seen by some as a set of policies geared to propagate materialism across the nation. The disgust of educated liberals, southern democrats, burned business partners, and alienated elites was, however, no match for the fervor of his supporters: Thaksin became the first prime minister in Thai history to complete a full four-year term in office, going on to win reelection in a landslide victory.

What to label Thaksin's governance strategy has been the subject of much debate in the intervening years. In CEO style, Thaksin vowed to run Thailand like a successful business. This included venture-capital type policies aimed at bringing more citizens, particularly the rural poor, into the market economy. It also involved the appointment of "CEO governors," who served to rein in the provinces that had grown increasingly autonomous as the result of a mass democracy movement's decentralization efforts during the 1990s.[15] Counter to dominant neoliberal strategy, Thaksin did create social welfare reform; but he was certainly not averse to trade liberalization (Glassman 2010). The state was heavily involved in orchestrating both market and social welfare schemes. Unlike the tripartite stabilization-liberalization-privatization platform heralded as the hallmark of neoliberalism, the Thai state actively managed domestic activities and the links between the domestic economy and the world economy. Thaksin promoted a "dual track," mixing capitalism and socialism and, in so doing, rapidly brought economic prosperity back to pre-crisis levels and beyond.[16]

Some find Thaksinomics an internally inconsistent and contradictory platform, riddled with buffoonery and corruption; others find it a coherent, albeit neoliberal, strategy. Unfortunately, scholars often have difficulty separating from their ideological stances to present an accurate depiction of this polarizing character and his policies. Claudio Sopranzetti (2013) strikes perhaps the best balance in likening Thaksin's governance to Chinese state capitalism, as well as to originary models of neoliberal governance, or what he calls "regulated neoliberalism." Microcredit, state-sponsored local business ventures, even universal healthcare—Thaksin's populist programs decreased the barriers to entry into the market economy for budding entrepreneurs by taking care of basic needs, swinging the doors of capitalism wide open.[17]

This all has relevance for the development of national policies for older people. Thaksin's populist programs created an opportunity, at least indirectly, for elder-care advocates to push for greater state support for older people. Pension programs for older people are a case in point. Following the introduction of universal health care, advocates for elders lobbied for universal pension schemes, including an expansion of the existing (but very limited) means-tested old age allowance program and greater access to contributory savings plans. With the urban and rural poor electorate as a new force to be reckoned with in the political landscape—that is, constituencies that actually expected policies enacted to benefit them—the governments that formed after Thaksin's ouster were compelled to maintain some semblance of populist programming. Democratic prime minister Abhisit Vejjajiva, for instance, introduced the 500 Baht Universal Pension Scheme in December 2009, which increased coverage for older people in need, and approved a national contributory public pension system (Thaworn Sakunphanit and Worawet Suwanrada 2011).[18]

But perhaps more than any money-transfer strategy, volunteer programs have come to define the core of Thailand's plan for older persons; and volunteer schemes, too, are caught up in political discord, from their funding and structure to the interpersonal relationships on which they rely. Volunteers have long made up a vital component of the Thai government's social welfare strategy across sectors, aging preparedness now included.[19] As discussed in chapter 4, the program Volunteers Caring for Older People at Home, or Aw Paw Saw (อพส), administered by the Ministry of Social Development and Human Security, was piloted in 2003, signed into nationwide law in 2007, and is now officially present in every district in the nation. It promises access to home-care support to all in need through the services of "friendly neighbors."

Formal volunteers have emerged as a central element in the shrinking of many social welfare states.[20] Andrea Muehlebach has shown, for instance, that the Italian state's promotion of volunteerism works hand in glove with neoliberal policies, functioning to mobilize free labor for the privatizing state. In particular, she traces therein "the creation of a new sense of self and good citizenship, of interiority and action, of sensitivity and agency" (Muehlebach 2012, 9). This emerges in Italy through the mobilization of Catholic imaginaries (in the "Catholicization of neoliberalism") and state-mediated norms of ethical sociality (and the "production of compassion"). Indeed, states around the world seem increasingly to support "governing through affect" (Rudnyckyj 2011)—efforts to promote or even induce particular affective and psychological states through workshops, role-plays, and other various "confessional technologies" (Nguyen 2010)—which seems to prompt individuals to take on the burden of family and community welfare, embody global economic competitiveness, and jockey for position in new resource distribution channels.[21] Analysis at the global scale shows volunteer programming allows states to legitimize privatization, renegotiate the social contract, and promulgate particular humanitarian platforms.

But volunteer programs in Thailand offer a powerful foil to analyses emerging from Western states. As I detail in subsequent chapters, similar processes of interiorization and ethical formation are on the rise in Thailand through volunteer training mechanisms. However, volunteerism interfaces differently with non-Christian modes of psychosocial support and long-standing sectarian debates that alter the stakes in Thai contexts. Confessional technologies are rooted in Christian norms of disclosure that appear increasingly in the form of verbalizing private, reflexive, psychological states (see Friesen 2017). But confessional technologies are not at the heart of most operating Thai logics. Whereas funding agencies and governmental policies around the globe propagate volunteer initiatives with similar formats, in Thailand these manifest in people's homes in relationship with karma, merit, and ritual formations in place. Examination of the original intent and the repurposing of volunteer programming offers a view into the dynamic interplay between—and indeed, the co-constitution of—intimate relations, structure, and power. Starting with care allows a view into the means by which social infrastructure can orient people's lives, as well as into the limits of structures alone to define experience.[22]

Indeed, care—the habituated actions of providing for others based on what counts in context—can alert us to how core social structures themselves emerge in and through habituated actions. Close examination of lived experience, at bedsides as readily as in conference rooms, offers unexpected theoretical openings into radical alterations of social formations, both those already occurring and those desired. But to bring them into view, one must suspend dominant ethical, political, and conceptual commitments and assumptions, even if just temporarily, to see alternate possibilities as they may arise.

A Critical Phenomenology of Care

This book is phenomenological, advancing what might be called critical phenomenology.[23] The range of uses and meanings of phenomenology in the social sciences is wide, but I invoke the phenomenological here primarily to bring focus to the social training of perceptual awareness and the lived experience that results from such ingrained attention to the world, both inside and out. I build on a long tradition of phenomenological anthropology (see Desjarlais and Throop 2011 for a helpful review). In continental philosophy, phenomenology is a lineage founded in the early twentieth century by Edmund Husserl. Husserl sought to confront and investigate the "anonymous subjectivity" presumed by the natural sciences, the roots of which he felt were poorly understood.[24] "Bracketing" (or the "phenomenological epoché") was conceived as a trained process of suspending judgments about the world from our programmed or preconceived "natural attitude" in order to apprehend subjective experience. Rather than accepting this method at face value, I take it as a cue to home in on the processes by which human attention is trained in the social world. Perhaps one could say I seek analysis of "natural attitudes" themselves. Such attention in particular Thai contexts serves to decenter dominant Christian and Euro-American ideas about care, providing a new vantage point from which to consider ritual and morality, and social change as well.

I begin with the simple contention that there is a great deal to gain from recognizing the ritual aspects of care. This seemingly straightforward statement belies the long and fractious history of ritual studies, including the extensive ripple effects of the Protestant Reformation's verdict on ritual.[25] By ritual, I mean repetitive acts that achieve effects through their correct performance, rather than from any particular internal orientation to the tasks. This is illustrated in chapter 1 through the details of ordinary caregiving routines, combined with the importance of karma (*kam*) and merit (*bun*) for local understandings of care. These terms, karma and merit, reflect a robust understanding of cause and effect across lifetimes, in which showing up and doing the right actions are essential. I trace the connection between care and karma to highlight the importance of how people go through the motions of care, and how and why little emphasis is placed on directly cultivating inner orientations, even though equanimity is of central moral import. The details of embodied practices themselves help bring to the fore what counts, in context, as providing for others, which in turn provides a sense of the logics that come to define a place and its people.

This type of ritual framework invites an excavation of care in practice that lays bare unexamined contingencies in contemporary investigations not only of care, but also of moral agency and subjectivity more broadly. Contemporary scholars often take for granted that what counts most in care is the active intention to help.[26] Caring acts are understood to express intention, giving moral motivation and justification to these actions. This book disrupts a too-facile connection between care and intention. It is not that intent does not matter in Thailand. But in *Rituals of Care*, I show the ways in which showing up and performing care acts has tremendous moral significance and can harness great transformative potential as well.

Leading feminist literature places care at the heart of moral practice, often with a similar focus on care in action and doing.[27] Such work, however, is often squarely set in Western contexts or is explicitly speculative, without ethnographic engagement and related non-Western philosophical traditions to sustain new interventions.[28] I seek at once to build on and counter these trends with a focus on patterned, embodied modes of being for analysis of everyday moral action and the locally relevant traditions that undergird them.

The discussion of "rituals of care" in chapter 1 eschews prioritization of internal orientation and thereby upsets common presumptions about the internal correlates of care, but in chapter 2 I move on to investigate directly the place of intention and emotion in forms of care common in Thai contexts. While existing literature, particularly that led by Michel Foucault, might suggest a turn to modes of interiority and "technologies of the self" to make sense of these internal and affective registers, I show the limits of the particularities Foucault presented from the Christian hermeneutic tradition when applied to Thai contexts. For one, a fixed, individuated, internal self as focus of moral action seems out of step with core logics of the everyday practices I document. An alternate set of reference points is needed.

I therefore turn to fifth-century Pali philosophy and local understandings of the mind for help in parsing common forms of psychosocial support in contemporary Thai contexts.[29] The Pali Canon is the tripartite set of texts (or "baskets") that constitute the textual core of Theravada Buddhism, the overarching religion claimed by roughly 93 percent of Thais.[30] The Canon includes sermons of the Buddha (Suttas), a code of conduct for monks (Vinaya), and an in-depth treatise on the mind (Abhidhamma). The fifth-century figure Buddhaghosa remains one of the most notable commentators on this core set of texts. And Maria Heim (2014) has rendered Buddhaghosa's work accessible anew as a philosophical system, which I find offers much guidance for making sense of lived experience in contemporary Thai contexts. I am thus arguing for common sense at play in Thai social worlds, reflecting what Heim calls the "moral phenomenology" of Buddhaghosa—a prescribed training of awareness toward the soteriological goal of liberation from suffering—which serves to prime people's lived experience of the world. Whether or not people explicitly reference these philosophical or religious tenets, this logic undergirds common forms of interpersonal support. I am not claiming doctrine as ethnographic fact at face value; rather, I bring Buddhaghosa's theory to bear on contemporary experience, allowing it to do analytical work in bringing to light common ways of understanding the world and engaging with it.[31]

The basic components of "mind" are identified in the Abhidhamma as individuated entities, which are bundled together in any given instance to constitute experience. That is to say, mind is an umbrella term for the many parts that come together in various combinations.[32] The Abhidhamma consists of seemingly endless lists of these mental factors and functions—from sensory contact and conscious awareness to myriad forms of pleasure and energy—a daunting challenge for anyone wishing to map and master its content. Instead of scoffing at the lists as some remnant of failed taxonomical rationality, Heim shows that the form as well as the content of the manual are vital to its comprehensibility. That these various factors appear across lists and in reference to different phenomena reflects the many ways in which mental factors can come together. The combinations—the arrangement of these building blocks of experience—are seemingly infinite, depending on circumstances.

Habit can be understood from these philosophical tenets as a fundamental influence on experience, a constitutive force to be appreciated and manipulated. As the "mind" draws together component elements in an endless array of richly textured combinations, the composition of the mind is both active and passive, with past actions determining which combinations are possible in any given instance. Conditioning is an essential element of human experience and action, and karma sets certain parameters for experiential combinations. What's more, the social world elicits certain patterns with greater frequency, shrouding the ever-changing processual unfolding of existence with a powerful illusion of continuity. In this way, in this Abhidhammic theory of mind, intention and experience alike are necessarily and fundamentally affected by karma, routine, and the influence of others. Thus it is important to note that intention—that which classically anchors conscious choice and arguably enables motivating desires, as well as that which forms the basis of sincerity in post-Reformation Protestantism—is not considered in isolation in Pali sources or in most Thai people's casual consideration. Intention is but one part among many, making habit a strong component of moral agency.

I document elements of Thai social worlds that facilitate the training of awareness to confirm the presumed truth of impermanence. High-arousal emotions, for instance, are understood as fleeting, necessarily containing seeds of karmic baggage to be overcome. One can thereby appreciate the value placed on equanimity, as well as the social norm of distracting from or displacing emotional distress. As detailed in chapter 2, common forms of psychosocial support across Thailand intimately relate to this Abhidhammic theory of mind. Analyzing intra- and interpersonal care based on an understanding of mind as agentive in isolation or in concert with so-called hydraulic modes of therapeutic disclosure (such as when emotions are understood as building up under the surface, needing periodic release lest a flood ensue) would be an injustice to the sophistication with which many Thai people orient to the world and provide for others.

Understanding this orientation is vital for understanding care as moral practice in both personal and political realms. When dealing with morality, as with ritual, I seek to bring attention to habituated patterns. This is in step with many anthropologists who claim that unconscious or otherwise routinized actions embody social values, as much as any public or institutional articulation of right and wrong. However, despite such declarations, ethnographic attention is still paid largely to moments of contention and/or reflection.[33] Indeed, a focus on reflective moments regularly trumps elucidation of the more mundane, habituated instantiations of moral action. Veena Das has expressed frustration along similar lines, noting, "Because of the strong emphasis on intentionality and agency in our contemplation of ethics, habitual actions are often reduced to 'mere behavior'" (Das 2012, 139).[34] I therefore bring the Abhidhammic theory of mind that decenters intention into conversation with a wide swath of literature—from classic social science and continental phenomenology to cognitive science—to argue that moral agency can productively be understood as a function of habits of perception, which are themselves conditioned by social practice. With habit thus figured as part and parcel of moral action, a new terrain of moral modes comes into view.

In chapter 3, I apply this sensitivity to the social training of habituated awareness to the analysis of care in social groups. Here I look to everyday life in concert with others. From small community gatherings to conference plenaries, from workshop training sessions to the tenets of national edicts, I home in on the subtle cues taken regarding designated leaders of any given assembly. I mark steps taken to ensure group cohesion, along with the felt necessity of doing so. What I call "care of the social body" is undergirded by trained perceptual patterning that primes people to perceive themselves as part of a collective and to provide for the maintenance of certain forms therein, just as they would care for their own body's health and well-being.

This kind of appreciation of care in practice invites reassessment of common working assumptions at multiple scales of analysis. In chapter 4, I turn to those who volunteer for older people to examine means of providing for others in the civic landscape. What volunteers are presumed and promoted to be doing, as well as what they actually do, reflects a complicated terrain of competing karmic framings of care. For some, transfer of merit is achieved by rituals of care that rarely involve physical caregiving. Personal motivation is here seldom highlighted. A wide swath of volunteer programming maintains a familiar pattern of action on behalf of the less fortunate through preset or prescribed deeds. Others—including key organizations working for change in end-of-life care in the country—are promoting a "new" orientation for volunteering (*čhit`āsā*, or the spirit of volunteering), in which personal motivations and pro-social action offer a civic-engagement route to making merit and offsetting negative karma. There are power struggles over what counts as beneficial action in this regard. But underlying all seems to be an enduring ethical map based on merit and karma in a hierarchical worldview, karmic politics that continue to guide volunteer work and civic action in many guises.

In chapter 5, I pose questions of structural violence and stasis in relation to the hierarchy and habituation in various forms of care.[35] In many powerful analyses, structural violence is the term given to systematic limits placed on individual agency. This naming has served to illuminate systems of oppression and inequality. And yet, notions of individual agency, like intention, emerge differently in different historical and philosophical traditions. I show how Thai social worlds habituate people to feel themselves as part of collectives and to provide for one another through maintaining differentiated roles within groups, which forces us to consider anew people's complicity with repressive social forms. That is, we must reckon with the forms of care that emerge in and sustain oppression. Compassion and pity can thus come into view as two sides of what may be the same coin, with implications for humanitarianism beyond the borders of Thailand. Limitations are placed on individual agency in a multitude of ways in contemporary Thai society. The stakes of altering norms are high because care is enacted through patronage and patterned into micro- and macrostructures. Throughout my fieldwork, new models appeared to be arising, spaces opening within social bodies for people to individuate in new ways, including space to voice complaints where previously they may have held silent. Many observers predicted at that point that revolution was certain, that the repression of old forms had become ideologically opposed by the masses and would soon topple. And then the military staged a coup, and opposition fell largely silent. Paradoxes of care may be one reason why.

Plodding the Revolution

Pathways for overthrowing domination must, it seems to me, habituate people to provide for themselves and one another in new ways. If Riccardo Ciavolella and Stephano Boni (2015) are correct in asserting that "only if there is a radical cultural shift in everyday practices can political transformations be achieved" (5), I argue that one must appreciate the care felt in and imparted by everyday practices.[36] Embodied hierarchy in Thailand comes into focus in the pages that follow as a form of care. Moreover, social norms of providing for others seem to resubstantiate set relations at every turn. Yet changes are always afoot. Looking to everyday habits as a form of moral agency, I suggest a bridge between the immediacy of individual actions and the seemingly more static elements of social structure. As Brahinsky (2018) asks, "What comprises a more powerful agent for change: a singular moment, or a deeply sedimented sensibility or habit?" Thai caregiving contexts provide rich ground for understanding the hierarchical and ritualistic components of mutual aid and moral life as lived, as well as clues as to how transformation can occur at individual and collective scales.

Though quieted under military rule, street demonstrations have been part of the political process for decades in Thailand. One could certainly say such mass gatherings spark identity (re)formations and alliances, key to social change movements (Edelman 2001). But, giving care its due, the modes and motivations of such participation deserve open consideration. In Thailand, demonstrations are conducted within a commonsense framework that follows hierarchical cues and often sidesteps demands for "authenticity." To be clear, these protests reflect individual commitments as well as fuel passions, rather than simply amplify the ideas of group leaders. Indeed, despite accusations that people participated only in exchange for payment, Red Shirt protesters in 2009 and 2010 repeatedly asserted that they came to marches and street takeovers their own damn selves (*gu ma eng!*).[37] Nonetheless, taking cues from rituals of care, we can also appreciate what is imputed through people just showing up on the street, over and above any internal orientation to participation. This matters particularly at this historical moment because of the increased focus on subject formation from the ranks of social activists. In Eastern European contexts, for example, Maple Razsa (2015) finds support for new alter-globalization efforts seizing control not of the means of production in a Marxist sense but, rather, the means of production of the self. In the end, I suggest that looking beyond the Christian hermeneutical tradition of self-formation to more ritually inflected, passively conditioned components of self like that of the Pali tradition could provide a radical offering for global social movements from an otherwise conservative and authoritarian social world.

If we take seriously that intention has active and passive elements, we can see anew the import of cultivating habituated actions of body, speech, and mind. Much of what one does is a kind of plodding along. But in fact revolutions occur. Some have gone so far as saying they are always a surprise (see Bayat 2013). Seen from the ecological orientation of Abhidhammic philosophy, this makes sense, for the addition or subtraction of even one small element can pivot one state into another. What follows is an attempt to alert us to the plodding along in contemporary Thailand, as well as to subtle shifts in people's plodding. The priorities of what counts most as providing for others could just tip the scales toward embodying something new.

1

THE KARMA OF CARE
Ordinary Actions and Their Consequences

Ek appears at the top of the landing and gingerly descends the polished wood steps, his broad shoulders and back straight as he balances the small frame of his eighty-five-year-old mother-in-law, who lies, wrapped in a Chinese-style red satin blanket, draped over his arms. He passes quickly through his wife's sewing shop, which occupies the first floor of their three-story Chiang Mai shop house, through the glass door façade, and down to the pickup truck out front. Pillows line the flatbed of the old vehicle, waiting to take the old woman to her scheduled appointment at the district hospital. Ek exchanges a few jokes, heavy with political undertones, with his brother-in-law as their wives make a few final adjustments to the makeshift traveling bed. There is a brief reconfirmation of the trip's expected timeline (8 p.m. return if everything goes smoothly, much later if a blood transfusion is required). Room is made in the cab for the anthropologist tagging along. And then the monthly caravan is off, the old woman in the back with one of her daughters and her daughter-in-law, her eldest son at the wheel.

What do Aom, the old woman's eldest daughter, and Ek, Aom's husband, do while the others are gone? Aom sits back down to her sewing table, Ek heads back out to his garden plot, or they spend some time with their thirteen-year-old daughter, Nok, enjoying the now rare time they have as a nuclear family alone. Do they cherish this time? Do they feel a relief as the truck pulls away and leaves them without the immediate burden of care for these short hours? I am left only to imagine, for my questions later will most often be met with laughter and vague answers about how it is they continue with everyday work.

Certainly, there is always work to do. It seems never to end. Aom and her sister Ying are up every morning at daybreak. Soon they will sweep the house from top to bottom, spray and wipe the front glass, clean the stoop, water the plants, do the laundry, and begin lunch preparations. But, first, the faucets must be turned on, allowing water up to the second floor bathroom, where buckets are prepared for their mother's morning bath. There, on a low wooden platform on the far left side of the room, their mother has lain, save for the monthly trips to the hospital, for nearly three years.

The room is sparsely furnished—the bed, a log table with four wooden benches crowded around it by the window facing the street, a desktop computer on the far right by the stairs, and a glass wardrobe with samples of Aom's fashionable creations from earlier in her career as a seamstress. The motor of the air mattress provides a constant hum day and night, sometimes accompanied by syncopated rhythms from the overhead fans. The center of the room is empty, providing space for the tables, supply bins, and buckets brought to the old woman's bedside four times a day, as well as space for Ying's bedding each night.

When Tatsanii—also known as Yāi or Khun Yāi, meaning grandmother—first became ill, the room was filled. Aom, Ying, their younger sister Kannikar, Kannikar's two young children, and several aunts and cousins all made their bed around the family's matriarch. The air was jovial, and the gathered women spent the nights talking and often laughing, sharing the new tasks of caregiving and the merit gained by such work. They were perhaps all waiting for the anticipated, the inevitable, the passing of the beloved elder.

The story is a familiar one in Northern Thailand, as elsewhere. Tatsanii was a talkative eighty-three-year-old, involved in her neighborhood and busy keeping tabs on her ten children and running the family compound with her husband. One morning, she fell and began convulsing. The family rushed her to the hospital. As her body contorted, her right side bending at the knee, wrist, and elbow, the medical staff sent a tube down her nose to provide her nutrients. After she had spent weeks as an in-patient, the medical team packed her up and, with some instructions for her daughters, sent her home. Ek generously offered to lodge Tatsanii on the second floor of their home, a modern concrete dwelling built next to Tatsanii's old wooden house on the urban outskirts of the Chiang Mai municipal area. So there she went, and there she stayed. And stayed.

When I first met her family, Tatsanii had already been in a coma for over two years, fitted with a feeding tube, permanently bent at the knees and elbows, requiring a host of interventions each day.[1] The tasks are formidable, though Aom and Ying have gotten quite efficient over the years. In the early days, the basic routine—bathing, diapering, turning, propping, stretching, powdering, massaging, medicating, feeding, and so on—took three hours to complete. Now it takes the pair one hour to finish: one hour, that is, four times a day. And that does not include the laundry, the meal preparation, the house cleaning, the monthly trips to the hospital, Aom's work as a seamstress and mother, and all the unexpected bits of daily life that intervene.

With Ying and Aom as guides, in this chapter I provide a phenomenological account of the everyday tasks of long-term caregiving in Northern Thailand. That is, I attempt to give a sense of how people experience the circumstances described. As noted in the introduction, the phenomenological orientation of this book is geared toward the social training of perceptual awareness and the lived experience that results from such attention to the world. Here I bring attention, first, to habituated physical procedures: what is done day in and day out. I then show how the karmic framework in which these routines are ensconced allows us to productively understand physical care acts in terms of ritual: repetitive practices that achieve effects through their correct performance, rather than through internal orientation to the tasks. Ideal internal orientation (in the form of equanimity) and the moral salience of intentionality are the focus of chapter 2, in which I explore the philosophical tenets of the Abhidhamma and its emphasis on abandoning or refraining from, rather than cultivating, particular mind-sets. But here, to escape the pull of the dominant analysis of self-cultivation in the Western tradition, I emphasize the physical and show how awareness is trained on and with physical action. The details of embodied practice help bring to the fore what counts in context as providing for others. In turn, the "rituals of care" presented in this case upset common presumptions about the psychological correlates of care dominant in the Western tradition.

Care in the Field

What exactly happens, on the ground, in caregiving situations? How do caregivers conceive of their roles and take to their tasks? What is at stake for people as their everyday lives are reoriented by caregiving? How do people meet the often conflicting demands on their time and identity in the face of providing care full time? To answer these questions, I turn to Aom and Ying as examples of the many people—mostly daughters and wives, but also sons and in-laws and various next of kin—who perform the duties of family caregiving for their elders in a rapidly aging Thai society.[2] Their lived experience provides a critical contribution to our current assessments of care.

The term "care"—in the literature of nursing, medicine, philosophy, feminist ethics, and the like—generally hinges on an understanding of "caring" as an internal conviction, a presence of mind and body that is attuned to the needs of others. In this way, care is but one part of medicine's "dual discourse," the other part being competence (Good 1995; Good and Good 1993). By extension, people are thought to enact true or ideal caregiving when they attend to physical and emotional needs with (or because of) empathy, bringing about a communion meaningful to all parties involved. Thus analysts distinguish between "technicians" and "practitioners," the former being professional caregivers who fail to bring appropriate attentiveness and sincerity to their craft (Benner 1994, 58). Robert Bellah (1994) casts such a division as a "crisis" in the US health-care system, one whose deleterious effects require a great deal of energy to counteract.

But is this conception of "caring" a universal way of understanding the role and experience of the caregiver? Or are there particular sets of emotional and practical ways of being with people, ways with specific historical lineages, that can be differentiated as care in various contexts? I affirm different modes of care, and this chapter begins the unraveling of the lineages operating in the Northern Thai context that underlie not only processes of care but also more general understandings of the self, subjectivity, morality, and social dynamics.

Although anthropologists have long been interested in care-related topics—from the culture of biomedicine to the invisibility of home-care work, from humanitarian intervention to indigenous healing practices—it is increasingly clear that care itself has been undertheorized. Medical anthropologists have recently renewed attention to care and created space for a more comprehensive discussion.[3] But all too often, anthropological work glosses over embodied practices, prioritizing other analytic concerns—such as emerging technologies of the self and subject formation, health-care professionalization, and social welfare reform—or simply transforming the mundane into something considered worthy of inquiry.[4] And although there are important exceptions,[5] ethnographic inquiry into embodied care practices outside European, North American, or predominantly Christian contexts is limited.[6] Perhaps as a result, many analyses overdetermine the concept of care—particularly in relation to the often implicit connection that authors make between distinct inner states, among them beliefs and intentions, on the one hand, and outward actions and expressions, on the other. To unlock care's potential as an object of study, it is necessary to revisit these analyses' assumptions, which are evident in their emphases.

Take the emphasis on ethical reflections as a window onto the moral aspects of care.[7] Julie Livingston and Arthur Kleinman, for example, both demonstrate how caregiving is a profoundly "humanizing" moral act, but their reliance on ethical explanations and justifications obscures the insight, from the anthropology of morality, that the mainstay of ethical life lies in habituated activity.[8] Livingston (2012) powerfully argues that nurses in a Botswana cancer ward rehumanize their patients by normalizing physical conditions that elicit disgust in others. Yet she does not fully distinguish the habituated care routines that allow these nurses to act in such a manner from the nurses' Christian-inflected ethical claims about their behavior; in turn, context-specific orientations to care work become naturalized as part and parcel of rote action.[9] Similarly, while Kleinman's "notion of a divided self with hidden values" (2011, 805) provides a vital rallying cry for self-reflection in biomedical caregiving, such an evocation of care in other contexts may too quickly map a presumed set of universal orientations to care onto what Michel Foucault (1988) traced as a specifically modern Christian hermeneutics of the self.

Another emphasis in ethnographies of care has been the irreducibility of care to economic considerations. Such work seeks to maintain a distinct relational space for care, even while acknowledging the effects of economic pressures and sociopolitical conditions on the working conditions of care. This emphasis could establish a more robust understanding of care in practice, but, I would argue, only if combined with attention to ordinary embodied experience. Upholding a simple opposition between care and commodity leaves open the possibility of misprescribing particular emotional or cognitive components as if they were intrinsic to the category of care universally (Zelizer 2010). Even if we maintain, following João Biehl (2012), that care is not a commodifiable or technological intervention but a "relational practice," we still need to investigate how people constitute such relational practices across contexts.

Studies of the political uses of care show a similar propensity. Following suit, one could argue that the political logics of long-term care mirror those of humanitarian discourse as a whole—insofar as caregivers are cast as victims, erasing the political and economic causes of their suffering and requiring particular performances of distress for aid (Fassin 2012b; Ticktin 2011). But for such an account, the underlying orientation and practical daily affairs of such "victims" need barely surface. Paying close attention to people's embodied experience, like that of Aom and Ying, could reinfuse political and economic analyses with a sense of what is changed and what is lost sight of in the wake of social and economic reform aimed specifically at care.

In short, the scholarship on care currently misses the possibility that care can be separated from particular psychological states and correct intentions, and can in turn be productively understood in terms of physical practice or, as I argue, as ritual. Conceptualizing care as ritual allows us to get beyond meaning-centered approaches that presume that physical acts and core sincerity are aligned in cases of "real care," and to concentrate on what counts most in context.[10] Moreover, it allows us to pay attention to what caregivers do rather than just what they say they do, substantiating moral life as lived. And it brings us closer to the heart of anthropology, where discursive analysis is less important than "being there" (Borneman and Hammoudi 2009). Just as Talal Asad (1993) brought attention to the importance of practice over the uncritical privileging of a narrow conception of belief in religious studies, so too should we call on care studies to delve more fully into embodied routines.[11] In doing so, we can productively explore care as habituated action separated from internal orientation, at least provisionally, to bring a wider range of human experience into view.

Many factors—including economic status, profession, family and community makeup, accessibility of health care, and so forth—contribute to the composition and duration of the daily tasks I describe in the pages that follow. Aom and Ying are neither desperately poor nor solidly middle class. They represent a demographic in decline—those with a large sibling base to share the physical and financial responsibilities of caring for their mother. Aom's home-based business and Ying's unemployment make their physical care more reliable than that of people who work outside the home or cannot support an unemployed household member. People who are better off often employ help or stop working to free up caregiving time; those without such resources often cut corners in care or fall into more difficult circumstances as a result of maintaining home responsibilities. The Thai universal care plan has in recent years broadened health-care access nationally, but without all-encompassing provisions for home aides, it does little to diminish the physical demands of long-term dependency.

These factors contribute to one's phenomenological orientation to such tasks. But overcontextualization along these lines risks eschewing the point that, regardless of who performs these duties and in what circumstances, people do physical work to maintain other bodies. Describing routines shows how care lies in habituated activities and suggests that we can look to the patterning and embodiment of habituated actions in general to understand what values people enact and how they maintain social worlds through the physical practices of providing for others. Only with attention to the mundane, the banal, the everyday can we provide a robust basis for investigation and cross-cultural comparison; without such attention, we risk overdetermining the values, psychological makeup, and structural influences on the embodied engagement that constitutes care in practice. Most importantly, what Aom and Ying represent is something subtler than a set of social and economic circumstances: their physical routine, rendered as ritual, provides insight into a lived reality that escapes dominant forms of referential meaning and instead brings to light important ways of being in and understanding the world.

Routines and Resemblances

The faces in the hospital alert you. Not the individuals, but the pairs, or those grouped in threes and fours. They sit in the chairs lining waiting rooms, often staring vacantly—the fixed look of those waiting for the unescapable, the unspeakable. There you see the same slope and shape of a nose repeated down the line, the same contour of face duplicated in mother and daughter, in father and son, in sisters patiently sitting together. Do the children look over to see a mirror of their futures in the wrinkles of their parents' faces?

Between Tatsanii and her children, it is harder to see the resemblances. Perhaps that is because she lies contracted and unmoving, with no clues from inherited gestures linking the generations. Or perhaps it is because I have become so intertwined with the family, after months of visits and interviews and meals and outings, that I miss their similarities, just like I cannot see the lines of my mother's face in my own, though everyone says they are there.

On this particular hospital visit, Ying is hovering over her mother's gurney. It seems both a protective and performative stance, eager as she is to play the primary caregiving daughter—and earn credit and respect for such a role. Hospital visits are fairly routine, and the family no longer questions the utility of going to see the doctor, if they ever did. We are waiting in a hallway, a slim corridor leading to an open window, with some doors into examination rooms scattered along the hall, waiting to be called into the neighboring emergency room for Tatsanii's feeding tube to be changed. As a foreigner, sometimes I am permitted to stand closer for this change than is usually allowed. In so doing, I try to glean some staff perspectives on her case. Could the family possibly change the tube themselves at home? (No, a nurse must do it.) Is there any program whatsoever that could provide home visits, sparing them the arduous trip to the hospital? (Some say "no," some say "yes, of course," followed by the list of public programs available, all of which have been petitioned to no avail.) Some practitioners are rougher than others. With a choke and a moan, the old discolored tube is yanked up and out— longer somehow than seems possible for this four-foot-long woman in the bed— and a new one inserted. In a flash, it is done, and I am left wondering why it was necessary to come.

There is one more task to complete before we can be dismissed. Our caravan— Ying; her eldest brother, Jidtuporn; Jidtuporn's wife, Dee; Tatsanii (or Khun Yāi) on her wheeled gurney; and I—proceed to another hallway to await the results of the blood tests. Tatsanii's blood had been hastily drawn when we first arrived, the nurse missing the vein several times before succeeding in bringing the burgundy liquid into her vial. Each time the needle flailed and missed its mark, the old woman's face puckered, and she moaned in the one deep-throated tone she is still able to produce. This moan haunts their house throughout the day and night, though often there is no direct correlation between some outside stimulus and Tatsanii's seeming complaint. But here, in the hospital, it is an uncanny reminder that this woman does hold some connection to our world, however difficult or painful that is to imagine.

Word finally arrives that the old woman needs a blood transfusion. I am taken aback. Even though I knew this happens fairly frequently, I had yet to witness it in person. What could be the use of putting this old body through such an intervention, I wonder. Moreover, why hasn't anyone in the family mentioned to the staff that Tatsanii has been sick with diarrhea for the last several days? Would that alter the decision to subject her to the hours it takes to infuse her with two bags of blood? I take it upon myself to talk with the nurses about the case. The eldest of the harried nurses in the small blood transfusion unit agrees to print out the details of Tatsanii's test results. It is vaguely explained to me that an iron deficiency prompts the procedure. But while there is no trouble procuring the blood necessary for this work, acquiring a designated bed among the privacy screens is another story: her bed is put against the wall near the nursing station and, once the nurses get back from break, Tatsanii is prepped there.

A flurry of activity ensues. Ying has insisted that the old woman needs to eat dinner; it is approaching 8 p.m. Jidtuporn appears with milk, and Ying finds a beaker to plug in to the feeding tube. Ying attaches the feeding apparatus and sends down two snack boxes of milk, one after the other. We straighten the red blanket from home over the woman's small frame, and then we head out, to eat some dinner ourselves, at a stall down the road a short walk from the hospital.

The mood is light along the way and throughout the meal. It is routine, and no one seems overly concerned. Once we are back at the hospital, we set up camp, so to speak, in the open-air lobby of the hospital's main entrance. Dozens of other families share the space among the connected rows of low-slung light-blue plastic chairs; nearly all eyes are turned upward to the televisions hung from above the cashier and pharmacy counters. The evening's most dramatic soap operas are on, and it is hard to tear my eyes away from the lovers' betrayals and supernatural visions to observe what is happening around us. A young pregnant woman in a long pink maternity dress slowly lowers into a nearby seat as her fresh-faced husband approaches the counters to fetch a bag of medications and settle their bill, while, on the screen above, a woman screams and falls to the ground. Behind our backs, lines of young white-coated attendants wait to assist those arriving by emergency vehicles or on makeshift beds like ours, fashioned in the backs of pickup trucks, just as the woman on TV is escorted to a homey hospital room on-screen.

Ying and I somehow tear ourselves away from the scene to check on Khun Yāi. She lies where we left her, under the bright glare of fluorescent lights glinting off her red satin covering. She is alone and unmonitored, but all seems well as the first bag of blood slowly drains into her arm. (Was there a faint smell of a dirtied diaper? I cannot be sure, and do not think about it too much, as I am feeling lazy and the prospect of changing a diaper strikes me as a major hassle.) I wonder if I would leave a friend or family member's bedside under such conditions in an American hospital (deciding most likely not), but the call to go with the flow (not to mention the soap's storyline) brings me back to the waiting room.

Back in the lobby, time passes. A soldier arrives, carried on a stretcher flanked by a raucous crew in camouflage fatigues. The TV drama takes a serious turn as a neatly manicured woman battles a ghost that only she can see in a shopping mall parking lot. Jidtuporn asks me about America, about salaries and working conditions. Jidtuporn's face is animated, a rounder and plumper version of Tatsanii's face. I wonder whether he has inherited his style of social engagement from her, or how the two of them might have interacted. We then meet another sister-in-law (who works at the hospital) and her child. They, too, chat with us jovially before departing for home. After they leave, Ying leans over and whispers conspiratorially of their backstory. This woman, now heading home, is in fact one of two of Ying's playboy brother's current wives. Perhaps so she can tell me juicy details, or perhaps just for a change of pace, Ying and I head back to check on her mother.

We joke down the corridors, she grabbing my hand to lead me the way we've tread now many times before. At first glance, everything seems status quo with Khun Yāi. But as we near her bed, I begin to smell the distinct odor of wet feces—not the strong but flat smell of solid waste, but rather the pungent tang of a sick bowel movement. My heart drops in my chest as I notice, even before we pull back the cover, dark stains seeping through patches of the bright red cloth.

It is a disaster. The old woman's body lies as usual, crimped at the elbows and knee in familiar fashion. It was a Tuesday, and Tatsanii had been neatly dressed according to the Thai astrological color of the day. Her light pink sleeveless rayon cotton shirt matched the darker tones of magenta in her paisley *phā thung* (a common rectangle of cloth worn as a skirt, like a sarong), both pressed earlier in the week by Ying, standing over the ironing board in the middle of their sewing shop. A small change purse with a few coins had been zipped into one of the side pockets of her blouse, in case she should pass away and need passage fare in the afterlife. Two flat adult diapers had been laid underneath her *phā thung* and folded together across her body, fastened with two giant safety pins, one at her hip, the other just above the bent knee. Like many in similar situations, the sisters have found that fastening a diaper around her crotch is awkward and ineffective, and in general this system allows for maximum coverage area, along with neatest presentation. But on this evening, perhaps nothing could have stopped the flood.

Her blouse is bunched up around the top of her skirt, wet and dark brown at the bottom edges. The smell overtakes me, and I choke a bit as I scan down her skirt, darkened patches evident at the folds, to her dainty bare feet, also now tinged with brown at the ankles.

My mind flashes to her milk dinner. Ying and I exchange looks as the situation sinks in and we spring to action. She scurries off to tell her brother and sister-in-law—together they go off to buy diapers, toilet paper, latex gloves, a plastic bowl for water, and soap solution—and all three return with remarkable speed. Ying and I turn Khun Yāi on her side, first left, then right, lifting the soiled shirt up and away from the lower half of her body. I gingerly undo the safety pins, putting them aside as Ying unpeels the skirt from her body. Again we rock her body to one side; this time, I hold Khun Yāi in place as Ying tries to fold up the soaked diapers and somehow wipe away all that is spattered across the old woman's backside, before placing a fresh diaper pad under her raised hip and then rolling her onto it to repeat the process on the other side.

Thai toilet tissue is somewhat rough and extremely thin; it crumbles and disintegrates in the water as we try first to wet it and then wipe the old woman's body. It seems an interminable prospect, but somehow we start to make headway. Dee stands tentatively at the side of the bed, intermittently offering her hands to help with the process. Later, she admits that was the first time she had seen Tatsanii's diaper changed. It is clearly a first for her husband Jidtuporn as well, as he orbits around the top of the bed in his full khaki military uniform, shifting his weight from side to side over his shiny black shoes. The serene and lighthearted expression he wore all day is now clouded, as a dent appears on his forehead just above and between his two eyes. He takes a kerchief out of his pocket to dab the gathering sweat at his temples—his eyes fixed in the direction of the bed yet, somehow, not quite focused. He tries to be engaged as best he can, approaching the bed at one point to readjust the old woman's head and plump her pillow. But for the most part, he stands back. It strikes me that his position is quite strategic: he is short, and standing six to eight feet away, he can observe without catching a glimpse of the breast or vagina of his mother's body, laid bare and vulnerable under the harsh hospital lights.

We finish, somehow. Jidtuporn and Dee are back in the hospital lobby, again seated under the comforting distraction of television soap operas. As Ying straightens up, I head to the lobby to try to gather reactions. Jidtuporn's face has returned to a more placid expression. Dee, seated beside him, is a bit blanched and much more willing to engage on the topic of what has just occurred. Her tone is disapproving, as she notes that the old woman really should be wearing pants. I am a bit surprised—it is as though she is suggesting that the mess could have been avoided had their diaper and clothing choices been different. In hindsight,

I realize, I too was preoccupied by my own judgments of the situation, convinced that it was a wrong move to give the old woman milk when she had been sick already for three days. Jidtuporn is largely silent, allowing his wife to complain for several minutes until he subtly draws the conversation to a close. On the car ride home, as the two of us sit alone in the truck's cab, I try again to elicit his emotional response to the night's events. He instead casts his reflections in Buddhist terms and talks generally about duties and merit, rather than about the disturbing realities of cleaning up feces.

Ritual Repetition, Karmic Coordinates

Nearly everyone I spoke with during my research talked about their caregiving situations in terms of "karma" (*kam*, กรรม) and "merit" (*bun*, บุญ).[12] Jidtuporn was no exception, answering my questions not with admission of emotional upset, as I expected, but with acceptance of the karma of their situation and the merit made by physically providing care. In the broadest sense, these terms relate to a theory of actions and their consequences across lifetimes.[13] Most Thai caregivers, particularly children caring for a parent, think of the caregiving relationship as one in which moral destiny plays out.[14] To be clear, these are people who often work in tandem with state-of-the-art medical care and who understand as well as any layperson disease categories and treatment protocols. Although it is common for Thai families to shield a terminally sick relative from their diagnosis and prognosis, this karmic logic does not replace a biomedical framework; however, the severity of suffering and the length of time from illness onset to recovery or death are generally understood to depend on the merit of the ill person and the karmic baggage of all those involved. Difficult caregiving situations might be the result of past misdeeds; by the same token, providing care allows people to accrue merit and to use up (*chai kam*) the ill effects of past actions. Thus the performance of care tasks both plays out one's fate and offers an opportunity to change it.

Simply put, karmic debts as well as seeds of merit span lifetimes, spirit worlds interact with that of humans, and human-made offerings can be transformed into tangible outcomes in other realms when someone shows up and goes through the motions of set ritual acts. In Buddhist temple settings, this logic is enacted when one goes to the temple "to make merit" (*tham bun*, ทำบุญ): the flowers, incense, and money one offers are transformed into effective karmic agents (or antidotes). Similarly, on the Northern Thai "day of the dead" (*salaakapat*, สลากภัต), when people donate clothes, food, and other items, the deceased can actually receive such things in whatever form appropriate to their own realm.[15] As Stanley Tambiah argues, using J. L. Austin's (1962) theory of performativity, these Thai practices are constitutive ritual acts—like marriage vows, baptism, or the christening of a ship. What is more, the *"perlocutionary* (functional) consequences" of such rites cannot be judged on the basis of "Western rationality" (Tambiah 1979, 135; emphasis original). So, although the effect of such rituals may be uncertain—one cannot determine whether one's dead grandfather received the razors and snack cakes or that one's merit has been increased—the rituals' performative validity stands. Similarly, flagging beliefs or doubts do not necessarily undermine their validity either.[16] Awareness is trained on the material preparations, one's physical comportment, doing the right things.

Jidtuporn's emphasis on karma when reflecting on the hospital scene invokes a connection to such performative rites, ubiquitous as they are in Thailand. This kind of ritual activity is performed correctly through the motions themselves, without the enforcement (or promotion) of "belief" in the process per se or a reflective orientation to the activity.[17] Symbolic or repetitious acts are capable of transformations across this worldly realm and otherworldly realms—even across those realms practitioners do not themselves try fully to comprehend. Whether or not we all had the karmic ramifications of our actions in mind, or even a wholesome devotion to Khun Yāi, our acts were having transformative effects. And as I argue in chapter 2, this is partially why emphasis is not continually brought to intention in key Thai settings; cultivation of different arenas (and ultimately abandoning intentionality) is necessary for escaping human suffering.

Arthur Kleinman articulates from his own experience the path most Thais I worked with took to becoming caregivers: "I learned to be a caregiver by doing it, because I had to do it; it was there to do" (2009, 293). Of course, rare is the caregiver who can articulate all they do in action. Moreover, what stands out as needing to be done can vary by cultural conditioning. This is life in the shadows of institutions, where "somatic modes of attention" (Csordas 1993) reign, officially suggested protocols find practical form, and meaning is caught in long-spun webs. How are we to make sense of these practical duties and everyday realities? What "counts" as care? Karma is part of the equation in this Thai context, but in what way? Could a "descent into the ordinary" (Das 2007) reveal truths (about bodies, about interpersonal relationships, about the purpose of actions) hidden in plain sight?[18]

Stanley Cavell marvels at the philosophical constructions that lead us to doubt insight rooted in ordinary experience. As he observes, "In philosophizing we turn the body into as it were an impenetrable integument" (1986, 97). Watching bodies bend over bedsides and relying on immersion in these gestures as a source of knowledge pushes back against this tendency in anthropological analyses. What do bodies giving and receiving in the most mundane circumstances show us, apart from all that we might want to project onto them? What values, what ways of knowing, what realities do their motions and pauses convey? Without retreating or escaping into analysis, is there a way to be present to what is occurring in direct view?

In an attempt to be present in this way, below I fully sketch a typical bathing. I deliberately drown the reader in detail to re-create the tedium, the repetition, the perfunctoriness that most importantly characterizes these daily tasks. I then work with the ritual frame of reference that permeates the local worlds of my Thai friends and associates to allow seemingly "hidden" aspects of their care practices to come into clearer focus. Arguing for care as ritual in this way allows for ambivalence and ambiguity in the analysis of caregiver experience, and also shows previously unexplored epistemic possibilities in an experience-near way. With conventional presumptions put on hold, goals of care and the means of accomplishing them emerge to reveal an important mode of relating to habituated actions, with reverberations across the social world.

Daily Practice: A Descent into the Ordinary

A long time passed before I assisted with washing and changing Tatsanii. For months I had watched the sisters perform these tasks and had even videotaped the process. It was not until my husband began taking sewing lessons from Aom that I was permitted to participate. The lesson on the first floor allowed me to head upstairs with Ying for the afternoon session.

Tatsanii's diaper is changed four times a day—in the early morning, midmorning, afternoon, and night—and she receives three meals (two with medication). A neatly handwritten sheet outlining the steps for each session remains taped to the wall over Tatsanii's bed, though its instructions are no longer needed, routine having long taken over. The early morning is the largest undertaking. The old woman usually defecates during the night, which brings out face masks and surgical gloves, along with the rest of the bathing accoutrements, a change of clothes, breakfast, and morning medications. The midmorning involves lunch and repositioning from one side to the other. The late afternoon brings another bath and her final meal of the day, followed by more medicines. At night, she is given one final change of diapers, and a mosquito net is placed over her bed to prepare her for "sleep."

First, preparation: Ying lays out a small pink floral plastic sheet on the floor and a larger one near the bed, later to be stretched underneath Khun Yāi. Next, two tables are placed on top of the first sheet, which will protect the floor from the inevitable bathwater spills. Additional materials are brought over—small plastic bins holding necessities like cotton balls, powder, lotion, and bedsore medicine. Then three plastic tubs are filled with water—one large and two smaller—and lifted onto the plastic floor sheet. Sometimes, a groggy silence permeates the scene; sometimes, a transistor radio is on, and the sisters remark on political events as they take to their tasks; sometimes, they are all thumbs, and laughter fills the air as bottles and basins tumble to the floor.

The second plastic sheet converts her air mattress into a bathtub. Then begins the process that will be repeated for all clothing and diaper changes, as well as all mattress adjustments—a series of rolling her to one side, shoving materials underneath her, rolling her to the other side, straightening, and easing her back to center. First, she is rolled to the right. Two people make this much easier; I might, for instance, hold Yāi on the right as Ying arranges the plastic protective sheet so that it is neat on the left and bunched up under the old woman. I roll Yāi over to Ying, who then holds her on the left as I straighten the plastic on the right side. It can take several rolls to get it completely straight—a meticulousness that seems gratuitous at first but decreases the likelihood of pooled water or, in the case of clothing or diapers, skin irritation. In a similar manner, we remove the old woman's skirt but leave the diaper for the time being, in case she urinates as we proceed.

We start with her eyes. The smallest tub—about the size of a soup bowl—is filled with plain water without soap. Cotton balls are soaked and used, one per eye, to clean the yellowish mucous from the old woman's eyelashes. The bud of the cotton ball makes contact, and on close inspection, sunken wrinkles part to reveal sparse encrusted lashes. If the eyelid opens enough with the movement, one might catch a glimpse of an eyeball rolling around, seemingly unseeing. The push must be gentle but with enough pressure to do the job. Here, the power of the back exerts itself in a new way: apart from the physical strength of lifting tubs of water, or lifting the old woman herself, or the constant bending to arrange materials, there is the strain of getting close enough to the small body, leaning across the bed to be effective but without breaking through the particleboard platform on which the air mattress sits. We balance our weight on the thin metal frame beneath the platform, careful to establish a solid base with enough power and control to maneuver through this delicate contact.

After wiping her face, we replace the tap water with drinking water in the small tub. More cotton balls are submerged, this time for the mouth. Ying brings a wet bud to Yāi's lips. Then, as with so many motions of this process, she begins a subtle bodily negotiation. She wipes across the lips, then begins to coax the jaw open, pushing the cotton in while encouraging Yāi to open her mouth. "Ah, ah, ah"— Ying makes sounds with her own mouth wide open, and, whether by the force of

Ying's fingers or by directive, the old woman's mouth opens, allowing her daughter to push the cotton inside to wipe her palate, the insides of her cheeks, her tongue.

We pat the old woman's now-clean face, neck, and ears with a dry cloth. Then Ying and I position ourselves on either side of the bed for exercise and massage tasks. With two caregivers, both sides are done simultaneously. In time, I will come to know that the right hand is tighter than the left, but the left arm is more diffi-cult to unbend at the elbow. First you bend the limb down and coax the elbow to release using a combination of calculated manipulation and sheer strength. The motion involves pushing the elbow down, bringing the hand across the body, pull-ing the shoulder out, and, finally, extending the arm from the elbow. If you hit the "sweet spot," so to speak, the elbow bends as if on cue; otherwise, real force is required. Once you lengthen the arm, you bring the hand into the body again by bending the elbow, and you repeat this, two, three, four, five, six, seven, eight, nine, ten times. Sometimes, you count aloud, numbers punctuating the conver-sation, unnoticed. Next, shoulder extensions, accomplished by bringing the fully extended arm out and up like a jumping jack, again ten times. Then, with the arm allowed to bend again, you massage the hand, gently bending it at the wrist and taking it through a series of circular motions in two directions, careful not to be scratched by the old woman's nails—ten times. Finally, on to the legs. The right leg is permanently bent at the knee and locked up. It is so thin, but again held bent with incredible strength. You have to massage the thigh and pull, despite crackling and crunching sounds, to straighten it out. This all entails a series of contortions, something like Thai massage, yoga, and weight lifting combined.

Here, as we stretch and straighten the legs ten times each, Ying might start com-menting on the difficulty of the work. "It's hard, *two*, *three*, isn't it? Lots of people say, *five*, *six*," and here she will not name names, "that it could be quicker. But unless you have physically done it, *nine*, *ten*, you just don't get it."

The washing begins. Rocking, propping, wiping, lathering, rinsing. One hand on a knee, the other alternating palm to back around the vagina. With chin hold-ing the bent knee or with the aid of a partner's hand, the belly flab is moved aside to access the hip fold. With practice, the tasks are effortless, and concentration can be light. Neck to toes. An unexpected urination, and the process starts again.

With Tatsanii washed and dried, it is time to massage with ointment. We pull out a tube of analgesic heat rub and dab a bit on our palms. Spreading it across our hands, we take an arm and spread the ointment the length of it, followed by stretching and massaging as before. Practiced movements help enormously, else you wind up doing a spotty job as you wrestle to get the limb untangled. We cover arms, legs, hands, and feet before we quit.

Powder helps keep things smooth. Perhaps we forget to apply the powder at first and instead go straight to putting on the diaper. Again we are rolling her to one side, arranging a set of two and a half diapers flat on the bed underneath her, and rolling her back. With the diapers laid down, the skirt comes back on. More turning and arranging, and we are set to affix the rectangular cloth skirt with two giant safety pins. Ying brings one corner of the skirt over to my side, and I take my corner across the waist to her end and, careful not to inadvertently attach the diaper, pin the skirt at the old woman's hip. We go on to start the trickier part of wrapping the sides down around the bent leg to pin the skirt in the middle, only then to realize we have forgotten the powder.

Off comes the skirt, and we are back to the bare limbs, powdering the legs, the hip crease, the armpits. "How nice and comfortable" (*Sabāi sabāi*, สบาย ๆ), coos Ying. Gently she puts powder on the old woman's face and, taking out a foundation pad to smooth it in, teases her mother for using makeup.

Then we are back to the skirt—rolling back and forth one more time. The trick is stretching out the bent leg so that, when one of us wraps the skirt around and pins it between the thighs, it will be held tight by the leg as it springs back into place. The diapers cover only the buttocks and down to the middle of the thigh. Gravity does its job most of the time to keep the skirt free of excrement, though every morning Tatsanii's clothes will be taken downstairs to another set of tubs for laundering.

Before we are through, we arrange the pillows that keep Yāi in place. Late afternoon is time to put her flat on her back. A duck-shaped pillow comes first. This and the other children's pillows may seem like an odd choice, or perhaps a chance reminder of the similarities between the very young and the very old, but they do in fact have their uses. The duck's bill is pulled through the woman's crotch to keep her legs separated. The bear is kept lengthwise, its head pulled between the legs to keep the separation down the limbs. Tweety Bird is put in service under Tatsanii's ankle to keep pressure off her heel. I cannot help laughing at the ludicrousness of it all. Finally, the regular bed pillow is placed under the woman's head, and her arms, now loose, are put under her back—soon to creep back up into their bent position under her red satin blanket.

Combing her hair is the last step. I brush her straight and soft white hair smooth against her skull, then tie it with a rubber band atop her head. I hesitate to use a straight rubber band, offering instead one of my cloth-covered hair ties—but of course, there is a reason to their method, and my offer is denied. Her hair is too thin and will not stay tied in cloth. The rubber pinches it tight, and we loop the hair at the end into a bun that will hold longer.

We begin the cleanup process as Aom's daughter climbs the steps with her grandmother's evening meal—a sienna-colored liquid blend of proteins and vegetables to be poured into a test tube attached to the end of her feeding tube. Upon completing our first session together, Ying assesses my reaction. "Is it hard?" (*Yāk mai?*, ยากไหม) she wants to know. I am not sure if she is assessing my stamina or trying to confirm how difficult these daily tasks are. Aom appears on the landing before I can answer. She is ready to mash up the evening drugs with a miniature mortar and pestle. These too will be deposited, mixed in water, into the test tube that, when raised, allows its contents to descend down the old woman's throat.

Overcome by what I have just experienced, I launch into a speech about how impressive their work is. Aom answers without blinking an eye: "Impressive? Come every day, four times a day, and *then* it will be impressive."

I took her invitation, living with the family toward the end of my fieldwork and sleeping at night on the floor beside the old woman's bed. In turn, my understanding of this impressiveness did pivot amid the repetitiousness of the physical engagement. And, beyond what Aom and Ying said, it was what they *did* that made clear both the implications of their explanations and the significance of their work.

Caregiving as Ritual

In contrast to dominant renderings of care centered on internal conviction, what I see emerging from the everyday realities of long-term caregiving is the fully embodied nature of care and care work. Bodies learn and perform the mundane activities of maintaining other bodies. Ying pushes with just the right strength, Aom bends and counts while listening to the radio, the sisters mount the stairs and perform their tasks in full again and again, with perfunctory rhythm and an automation in the repetition. These acts then can productively be understood as the routine action of ritual.

A ritual-based analysis can help disentangle acts of care from sentiment. Adam Seligman and colleagues (2008) provide a useful frame for such an analysis. These authors counter dominant trends in both anthropology and religious studies, echoing Catherine Bell (1992) with a focus on the "doing" of ritual rather than a search for its meanings. Through trained physicality, ritual creates a "subjunctive universe," a shared means by which people can reconcile disparate aspects of their lived experience through set actions (Seligman et al. 2008, 20–21). That is, ritual allows people a way of acting *as if* the world were a certain way, even when faced with uncertainty or contradictory evidence. A ritual mode of engaging the world then stands in contrast to a "sincere" or "authentic" frame, which demands coherence and consistency between belief and action (8). In ritual, the actions themselves, rather than internal cognitive orientations, are of utmost importance.

To argue that caregiving is ritual in this sense, we must overcome a "modern" or otherwise post-Reformation Christian tendency of equating "sincerity" with genuine enactment.[19] Too often, accounts of care take a "sincere" frame—as sketched at the start of the chapter, where an internal conviction is thought necessarily to underlie right action.[20] Presumptively emphasizing the "right" emotional or attentive orientation can lead us to minimize the importance of habituated routines to a moral life and to ignore the possibility that caregivers experience ambivalence. We can avoid these problems by using a ritual frame, which allows us to see how repetitive proceedings enact interpersonal, social, and symbolic functions by their performance alone.

In the karmic framework elucidated above, ritual acts function in the subjunctive. And although this orientation to ritual arguably includes a psychological element (as I explore in chapter 2), its contrast with a sincere correspondence between thought and deed is crucial. Through ritual, the ambiguities and ambivalences of life are assumed and accepted. Aom and Ying did not explicitly call what they were doing "ritual" (or what might be translated *phithī*, พิธี).[21] But in Thai, rituals are often called work (*ngān*, งาน) and are thus linguistically associated with everything from household chores (*ngān bān*, งานบ้าน) to cremations (*ngān phao sop*, งานเผาศพ) to weddings (*ngān tæng ngān*, งานแต่งงาน). Such linguistic association perhaps helps us bridge the gap (that scholarship may create) between the religious and the secular. Karma and merit can be seen in all aspects of life. A type of ritual work, then, can be done through caregiving, work by which one's karma is "used up" and merit is "made."

Ontological Pivots, Epistemic Possibilities

By the act itself, washing a mother's body changes the karmic coordinates of all the actors involved. This sharply contrasts with the mode of caregiving promoted in the humanist tradition of medical care, which, as noted above, often distinguishes between competence and care, and often presents care as depending on a particular correlation between inner states and outward actions. But in my ethnography, one witnesses the power of the action embedded in the physicality over and above one's mental orientation. A move away from referentiality—in which care is taken to mean a kind of internal caring—via ritual disrupts certain cognitive assumptions about care. It also provides a basis from which to gain greater specificity about competing influences on the lived experience of care in Thailand, and may offer insight about the lived experience of habituated action more broadly.

A tradition that conceives of the world as composed of generally untraceable roots, as is the case in these Thai conceptions of karma, helps reveal how ritual provides a physically embodied "as if" state that enables temporary coherence to the world. But this is not to suggest that karma provides the referential meaning behind my Thai friends' caregiving acts. Rather, the karmic framework helps dislodge the tendency to escape into analysis or otherwise seek analytical significance in cognitive explanations of physical acts. Paul Stoller (1984) provides a parallel when he draws attention to the power and importance of sound in Songhay cultural experience, arguing that he needed to *learn to hear* in order to recognize the force (rather than the meaning) of words. Ironically, it was the referential meaning of an incantation that alerted him to the importance of the sound itself; likewise, conceptualizations of karma and merit, and the correspondingly appropriate application of ritual, can teach us to appreciate physical action, extricated from valorized cognitive reflections that dominate analysis in a "sincere" or "authentic" frame.

Ritual and sincerity/authenticity are not the only modes by which people engage their worlds. Nor are they mutually exclusive. Spelling out their differences is, however, instructive, lest we inadvertently project a frame of sincerity onto ritual spaces. Scholars often analyze ritual by reading meaning into actions such that ideal participants are thought to be engaging with a coherent worldview actively in mind.[22] To suggest that belief is less important in ritual spaces than the actions themselves opens up new possibilities for analysis. This is not to reify a false dichotomy between mind and body, nor to draw too sharply the distinctions among what is said and felt and done; rather, it is to acknowledge that embodied practice can encompass an important range of possibilities.

More specifically, this ritual frame allows us to clarify the phenomenological realities of competing Buddhist practices in Northern Thailand—which as a whole are misleadingly cast altogether as Theravada Buddhism. Although the great majority of the people with whom I worked in Thailand self-identified as Buddhist (as does 93 percent of the country's population) and used Buddhist terms to describe their karmic burdens, their rituals of care do not fit a universal "Buddhist" mold. Going through the right motions is of utmost importance in one lineage of Thai tradition. But this calculus does not hold for everyone in Thailand. This overall depiction of ritual holds for the core of my particular interlocutors, particularly older people, those in lower socioeconomic classes, and those with less formal education.[23] Some Thais, however, maintain alternative configurations of "modern" or "cosmopolitan" Buddhism that challenge this type of ritual, cleansing what they find to be its "magical" elements to fit scientific, individuated, and sincerity-oriented claims on religious ritual and social practice which I explore in depth in later chapters.[24] Here, it suffices to call attention to a form of epistemic violence that occurs when, for instance, a well-dressed Thai woman whispers to me, at a temple funeral service rife with ritual activity, that "this is not *real* Buddhism."[25] For some, going through the motions of elaborated ritual is meritorious; for others, such ritual work is suspect as Buddhism (albeit perhaps comprehensible and efficacious in some sense nonetheless).

Both for this local case and in a broader sense, I argue that there is a danger in demanding emphasis on certain symbolic or meaning-centered coordinates of religious activities as well as of lay engagements—including caregiving. Doing so makes ontological presumptions that may not hold, or at least obscures alternative possibilities. The cosmos of continuous karmic interplay may be characterized as "chaotic" (to use the term of Seligman et al. 2008), or at least not a God-created singular world. Such ontological ground invites practitioners to act *as if* reality were one way in ritual actions, without necessarily understanding or presuming the cosmos *actually* maintains such parameters always. Because people in this context often use ritual activity to influence the course of life, linking caregiving to ritual does not, indeed must not, demand a "sincere" frame as the root of action.

In Northern Thailand, the term *tham fǭm* (ทำฟอร์ม) highlights elements of ambiguity permissible here. Borrowing from the English word *form*, one is said to "do" (*tham*) form, to act according to the established format. In those Thai settings where the "sincere" or "authentic" mode is more prevalent, *tham fǭm* is a derogatory phrase of sorts. But more often, one is in fact expected to do the form; following protocol is appropriate, regardless of one's inner relationship to the activity.

Showing up and doing the work of care is essential. In a daily cleaning session, one proceeds through the usual tasks; in a crisis, as in the hospital cleaning session, the familiar procedures take form as well. Rote routines make up the tasks of long-term care, and in fact expert care seems to demand a form of habituation. So while some theorists focus on instances in which people reflect on and challenge moral habitus to identify competing ethical norms and cultural shifts, the habituated core of quotidian life can serve a similar function.[26] Care can then be understood as *moral labor*—but not so much because of the ethical reflections that justify the work or the emotional attention that accompanies its back-aching forms. Rather, the repetitive forms of physical care work that populate any given day add up to the ethical whole, with mundane daily routines combined with their cultural significance providing a gestalt sense of moral life as lived.

Tatsanii is in an ambiguous state. Without medical intervention, she would have died years ago. Although she has a large family and thus several children who can share the enormous burden of providing and paying for her upkeep, Thailand's economic system makes such commitments increasingly difficult. Through a ritual framework, her family manages conflicting demands. Care occurs *physically* "in the subjunctive mode" (Good and Good 1994). By laying out the tables and drop cloths, preparing the water, applying the ointments, cooing the words, arranging the clothes, driving to the hospital, attending a blood transfusion, and so on, the family acts "as if" doctors were wise in placing the feeding tube down the old woman's throat, the sisters act "as if" their actions have some beneficial effect, and they all act "as if" their caregiving acts fulfill their dutiful roles as children—even if also receiving feedback from their own experience to the contrary. This is not a description of the meanings they ascribe to their actions at every turn. Ritual engagement provides an alternate way of parsing the burdens that emerge in this contemporary Thai context—a mode in which Tatsanii's caregivers are best able to negotiate their circumstances. It is how they care, and exploring this mode may shed new light on care in other contexts as well.[27]

"We Don't Need to Learn Theory—We Practice!"

Talking with Aom one day, I tried to get her to articulate more precisely her philosophy about merit and karma: how exactly people can "use up" karma and so forth. She began to answer but soon began to get jumbled. As her narrative broke down, she admitted, "It's difficult to talk with the vocabulary of dharma" (referring to the laws of nature as described by the Buddha). She stepped back and summarized: You are born into this life with karmic debts to pay, the roots of which cannot be traced. You might do "good" expecting to reap the rewards in this life, only to die and experience the benefits in the next. She went on to say that it is perhaps better not to think about these things, lest you rail against your situation or ask unanswerable questions. Finally, exasperated, she said, "Listen, we don't need to learn theory—we practice!"[28]

Aom is not thinking about karma and merit all the time. In fact, precisely what she thinks and believes is not prioritized as such. It is the actions themselves that count. Aom, and so many caregivers like her, is physically in the subjunctive: acting as if the world were this way, her caregiving actions making karmic transformations. She leaves the philosophical parsing and terminology to the monks and gives us a sense of how people perform these terms in the day-to-day: as motivations and justifications as needed, but largely in practice. Indeed, this "practice" or "field training"—the aspects of caregiving that in many ways defy verbalization—is essential to the particular sets of emotional and practical ways of being with people that count as care in this context.

So, on one level, "what counts" as care stems from bodies communicating and performing without a conscious cognitive component. Bodies can clearly do much more than the thinking mind is able to direct—in any context. Ying says, "Ah, ah, ah," soaked cotton poised at the ready, and Tatsanii's mouth opens—a seemingly spontaneous mimicry, the cause and effect hard to pinpoint. Work as a caregiver, or watch one work, and you will find bodies communing and engaging in a manner not easily formulated in words, and certainly not dependent on a steadfast affection or uncomplicated devotion. In another way, in this Thai context, transformations of merit and karma also "count," and here too, their particular lineage deemphasizes verbal articulation as well as internal sincerity in favor of technical achievement. For Aom and Ying, profound transformations occur without their conscious control. They value equanimity as they perform and complete their requisite tasks. One might even say they are simply and literally technicians of the sacred, "tinkering" (Mol, Moser, and Pols 2010) in the social world, attending to the gears so that the wheel of dharma can freely spin.

The Reach of Care

Rituals of care reflect how particular sets of emotional and practical ways of being with people can begin to be differentiated as care in different contexts. Many analyses of care seem instead to project a "sincere" frame of reference as universal. This Thai example provides a counterpoint that deemphasizes internal orientation in favor of the practical functions of caregiving—an emphasis on performance supported by cosmological formulations of karma and merit, and a lineage of Buddhist practice—which may provide new directions for the analysis of caregiver experience in other contexts as well.

Ritual analysis, as presented in this chapter, divorces caregiving from the shroud of culturally contingent sentiment—ideals of devotion, concern, intention, and so forth—and from the subtle transformation of habitual acts into representational forms that usually clouds the assessment of care. As Rosalind Morris contends, "When habitual acts are brought into consciousness and objectified, they are transformed; practice becomes representation, and everyday acts become strategies that presume a timeless and totalized vision" (1995, 583). When, instead, we take mundane, everyday routines as a source of insight about care, what "counts" in the context of caregiving emerges more clearly.

Care is a remarkable way in to embodied experience at multiple levels of analysis; however, it has yet to fulfill this promise because of assumptions snuck in under its rubric. Contemporary usage of the English word *care* may contribute to the tendency to assume a correspondence between particular internal states and the acts of best providing for another, or the parallel tendency to focus on ethical reflections about caregiving situations. *To care* can mean "to provide for" as well as "to feel affection for" or "to be concerned about"; contemporary definitions of *care* as a noun range from a type of caution, close attention, or attentive assistance to a burdened state of mind, mental suffering, or an object of worry. Someone who cares might be providing needed assistance or watchful supervision, be concerned or interested, or have a liking or attachment. Elements of concern, or feeling in general, are essential—thus a number of fields understandably define "true" and "meaningful" care as instrumental assistance coexistent with forms of mental and emotional attachment.

In Thai, the term *care* used in the situations I describe does not have the same multivalent definition. "To care" (*duulae*, ดูแล) is a compound of two words that both mean "to look." To care for another, to look after another, implies that the caregiver will heed their needs (*aojaisai*, เอาใจใส่). The emphasis is on seeing (perhaps even recognizing), with a connotation of guarding. My Thai friends explicitly denied that anguish, worry, or concern (*mai huang*, ไม่ห่วง) accompanied their acts of care. And although anxiety and "sincere" or active devotion arose, caregivers did not emphasize internal orientation as evidence of "good care," for reasons that will become clearer in the next chapter; rather, they viewed cleanliness, lack of bedsores, and other signs of physical competence as appropriate markers.

A focus on "rituals of care"—embodied routines and their accomplishments—allows space for caregivers' ambivalence. Such ambivalence does not indicate moral failing, as my case study makes startlingly clear. Instead, ambivalence—and even a kind of incoherence—seems appropriate, even necessary, for harnessing the energy to perform the work of care in a world of competing interests and enormous paradox. Rituals of care suture would-be wounds of ambivalence by acts of indeterminate correspondence. Precisely because care is free from an emphasis on the internal, caregiving acts can appropriately provide for others in a number of ways, making a moral life—and even the most profound transformations—possible. Perhaps contemporary experiences at bedsides everywhere could benefit from such conceptual space.

Overdetermined conceptualizations of care fail to provide ground on which to witness and address subtle changes afoot in the societies anthropologists study, when in fact care can and should be a robust tool for doing so. I contend that scholarship can assess the reach of, and individuals' articulation with, for instance, biopolitical incentives—in the form of increasing state reforms and various aid efforts—only once embodied experience is no longer assumed but recognized. Indeed, habituated actions of providing for others can be expanded from the individual and interpersonal level to the collective, for a fresh take on social organization and political change as well. I will continue to confine the definition of *care* to "providing for others" in order to open its potential as an object of study and analysis. Understanding what counts in context remains of paramount importance.

Here I have begun to replace presumptions of a set of universally relevant care attitudes, or the affect that animates them, with investigative work that unpacks such claims. Indeed, without such due diligence, analyses can quickly become normative rather than exploratory exercises.[29]

Understanding what people train their awareness on (and why) suggests how they experience the world, a phenomenological acuity that leads us to ponder questions that are more appropriately calibrated to local values. Here I have shown how crucial correct performance of physical tasks is. These actions also ideally share a predominant mood, one of equanimity or emotional calmness (*jai yen*, ใจเย็น). Restraint from overly emotional displays is also trained in Thai social worlds. In this way, values force and enforce particular patterns of habituated action and the presumed status of consciousness therein. Such distinct modes of providing for others can be linked to historical antecedents. A Pali philosophical tradition offers an important impetus for distinguishing among body, speech, and mind; in this chapter, rituals of care at the physical level have been separated out, to allow for the importance and particular forms of interdependence among body, speech, and mind to come into clearer view in the next chapter. In chapter 2, I turn to questions of intention, emotion, and self-formation from the vantage point of contemporary interpersonal norms in Thailand and their interestingly direct Pali antecedents.

THE CONDITIONING OF CARE
Intention, Emotion, and Restraint

On the car ride home from the hospital the night after Tatsanii's blood transfusion, Jidtuporn (Tatsanii's eldest son) reiterated what I had heard so many times before: caregiving is all about karma. A former monk, Jidtuporn spoke readily about the system of merit and karmic retribution at play in his family's situation. But in what might seem like a direct contradiction to my argument in chapter 1, Jidtuporn noted that people's inner orientation and emotional reactions to such situations were relevant, and that they were all about karma, too.

In chapter 1, I argued for an emphasis on the bodily components of caregiving. With care and karma closely linked, the physical practices of providing for others are important for settling debts and making merit in the karmic system of cause and effect. So what about interiority, intentionality, and affect? There are those who argue for the primacy of inner motivation in regard to ethical action and the creation of karma in Buddhist frameworks.[1] That is, what one *intends* for an action is thought to be what counts the most. And yet, among my Thai friends and interlocutors, very little (if any) attention was focused on directly cultivating intentions. There was no emphasis on cultivating a loving or compassionate or even "mindful" mind-set in relation to physical care acts. Likewise, there seemed no utility placed on sharing one's internal orientation, whether in regard to one's intentionality or one's emotional state. Instead, a type of placidity was favored. Indeed, even with an appreciation of the cultural construction of emotions, my expectations for caregiver sentiments and psychological priorities were confounded at nearly every turn.

I was, in many ways, primed to expect (or perhaps to desire?) a high degree of emotional sharing in my work with caregivers.[2] For one thing, the idea that it is healthy and important to share your feelings is prevalent in the American context—echoed as readily in children's programs as on talk shows and in mental health programs. "Letting it out," "blowing off steam," or "getting things off your chest" are all fairly common idioms that reflect this norm. Regardless of whether or not this idiomatic strain represents common practice, there certainly is no shortage of expert encouragement of emotional sharing. The importance of eliciting emotional expression is found in psychotherapy models, trauma research, and grief and bereavement studies, just to name a few. A recent National Cancer Institute booklet, *Caring for the Caregiver*, is a fairly typical case in point. Eight of its fifteen pages of text deal explicitly with feelings and the healthy (and necessary) ways of expressing one's emotions as a caregiver.[3]

My research soon confounded these expectations. Rarely did I encounter tears or confessionals as I worked alongside people dealing with major life events. I spent months upon months working with people arduously caring for infirm loved ones. I worked with volunteers who dedicated large portions of their time to helping dependent older people. As I describe in chapter 4, these volunteers readily shared information on health practices, presented gifts to older people and their families, and organized elaborate merit-making activities. But there was never much emotional talk, nor evidence of that talk occurring elsewhere.

What I encountered instead was support for external calmness and placidity, based on an alternative logic of interpersonal support. The forms of expression I found in context reflect what might be described as a "don't ask, don't tell" logic of psychosocial support. Admittedly, this at first struck me as a type of superficiality or closed-ness. But I have since come to appreciate these patterns in relation to a sophisticated local theory of mind tied to a philosophical tradition that predates Aristotle. Conventional restraints on asking and telling prompt distinct phenomenological states that deserve recognition, without presumption of an implicit underbelly of private turmoil held in or suppressed.[4] What's more, this logic's philosophical underpinnings challenge dominant models of mind and the self, models that, arguably, constrain studies in the social sciences at large.

So in this chapter, I turn attention inward, so to speak. I illustrate some of the emotional and affective states most evident in ordinary caregiving situations. To make sense of the patterns found there, I probe notions of intentionality, agency, and (non)self in the writings of Buddhaghosa, a fifth-century commentator on the Theravada Pali Canon. These notions, I argue, resonate with karmically inflected understandings of care at intra- and interpersonal levels in the contemporary world. In particular, I describe a Theravada "theory of mind" that distinguishes among acts of body, speech, and mind, but locates intention and karma in each.[5] By simultaneously collapsing and expanding the Cartesian mind-body dualism, this tradition indeed puts great importance on subjective experience as a key to wholesome karmic action; and yet, subjective experience itself is not the focus of cultivation. Internal orientation is not promoted or refined in ways one might come to expect through Western confessional "technologies of the self" (Foucault 1988).[6] Rather, this tradition guides people to refrain from certain actions and states, with ideal practices characterized by the absence of key defilements.[7] What reads at first as a holding in of, or a distraction from, painful emotional states ultimately reflects a highly developed and centuries-old moral psychology with incredible continuities evident throughout contemporary society.

In the discussion that follows, I characterize the gross contours of this logic as it surfaces in contemporary Thai society, and then I illustrate its manifestations in a typical end-of-life caregiving scenario. Buddhaghosa's commentaries on the Abhidhamma provide technical components of a Theravada lineage of thought, in which conditioning is an important factor in the composition of the mind at any given instance. This, in turn, helps us appreciate techniques for embodying values of calmness and acceptance and for recognizing efforts to acknowledge and manage the conditioning of experience. In light of this tradition, I discuss efforts under way to change common care practices, particularly in regard to emotional disclosure, and the implications of such efforts. I seek here to cultivate sensitivity to the multifaceted and dynamic Theravada lineage, and to utilize the theoretical tools its philosophical schools impart, to portray contemporary Thai social worlds with clarity and relevance for a richer comprehension of human subjectivities.

Don't Ask, Don't Tell: A Logic of Intra- and Interpersonal Support

The overall logic of the intra- and interpersonal support in question hinges on the notion that thoughts and emotions are transient. Distraction from or replacement of sadness or other unwelcome or unpleasant feelings is understood as a functional means to internal serenity. Mental states are necessarily temporary; letting them pass is the wisest way to handle them. In turn, the serenity and equanimity that results from such practice is a marker of religious attainment and moral virtue.

Some people put this logic in explicitly Buddhist terms. "Thoughts and emotions are fleeting," they say, echoing standard religious teachings. Just as meditation instructors remind their students, such people would remind me that we have a "monkey mind," which hops from topic to topic like a monkey from branch to branch. If you focus on a thought, you reinforce it. Thus, in recounting and re-hashing negative story lines (or "getting things off your chest," or "venting" to a friend), thinking about what you are most upset about is like throwing kerosene on a fire—you make it bigger and, in essence, more real. A friend, therefore, helps you take your mind off your troubles and helps you focus on something other than your worries, following teachings of impermanence.[8]

Others are less explicitly religious in parsing this logic. Jean, a recent college graduate and eldercare NGO intern, told me, "Your friend's job is to take your mind off things," not necessarily to engage in serious conversation about feelings. She went on to describe how her closest friend would, of course, know exactly how she was feeling without her having to say it directly. "We've known each other since we were two!" she exclaimed as explanation. A presumption of unspoken understanding, commonly evoked, seemed to suffice.

I sat one day with Jean and this closest friend she had mentioned, casually discussing such matters. Jean had been the primary caregiver for her grandmother for over a year—postponing college to change diapers, cook, clean, and care for her paternal grandma until the old woman's death. I was curious how her friend had supported her through that experience. Jean's friend reported that she could always tell what Jean was feeling and would respond appropriately—though she was unable to describe exactly *what* clued her in, whether tone of voice or topic of conversation or something else. The phenomenon was self-evident, as in the popular Thai idiom `ao jai khao mā sai jai rao (เอาใจเขามาใส่ใจเรา): simply trans-lated, "The wants and needs of others come into our heart."[9] But while this em-pathic capacity is taken as innate, what follows, or what should follow, is duty-bound according to cultural parameters. So, for Jean's friend, if she sensed Jean was sad or overwhelmed, she would suggest they go out shopping or to the movies. Would she engage Jean by talking about what was troubling her? No, not really.

I began this chapter, somewhat flippantly, calling this a "don't ask, don't tell" logic of psychosocial support: don't ask about emotional strife, because you should already understand it; don't tell others your woes, because the best way to get over heartache is to think about or do something else. And although there are partic-ular friendships in which emotional sharing is important, and certain individu-als who welcome such interaction from particular people, the general social common sense of "don't ask, don't tell" holds for overall public tenor and the general contours of emotional contemplation and disclosure.

There are personal and shared dangers of sharing emotional tumult accord-ing to this logic. Another Thai idiom helps illustrate the stakes: *fai nai yā nam`ǫk fai nǫk yā nam khao* (ไฟในอย่านำออก ไฟนอกอย่านำเข้า), which translates literally as, "The fire inside should not be let out, and the fire outside should not be brought in." In a general sense, the saying advises people to be humble, to hold things in, and to follow the top-down rules in a hierarchical system. Friends interpreted for me "the fire" in this phrase to be anything bad. "The bad inside, we don't express it. It is best to keep it inside yourself, inside your community, inside your organization. . . . Don't bring the bad to hurt people [others or yourself]." It is not that people never talk about their emotions; but the potential negative effects of such sharing are noteworthy.

One night, washing dinner dishes with Ying (the younger of Tatsanii's caretaker daughters), I got a lesson in these presumed effects. Ying was hovering over the sink as I washed, not exactly criticizing my efforts, but certainly taking control over the results. It was a typical dance of two "control freaks," an interactional pattern between us that often had me laughing at the ridiculousness of our moves, all while trying to take in everything that was passing between us.

"I could tell you a heartbreak story that would really make you sad," Ying told me, as she rearranged a couple of plates I had just laid on the drying rack. I told her that my heart was big, I could take it in—thinking that she was referring to her former husband who, as she had described to me weeks before, had left her for a younger woman she herself had first befriended. But Ying had other tales of woe in mind, including the untimely death of her main benefactors and the loss of her best friend who died while working in Singapore.

Part of me would like to claim that this evening's chat was an indication of our becoming *sanit* (สนิท), close friends who could share their troubles. That is, I would like to see proof of familiar strategies of intimacy in this interaction. But, in fact, Ying's stories were intertwined with subtle manipulations to elicit pity (and money) in addition to any genuine expressions of camaraderie. Furthermore, as Leela Bilmes notes, whereas "North Americans tend to use self-disclosure as a relational strategy to initiate personal relationship, . . . for a Thai, such a strategy would be rare, and for many unthinkable" (Bilmes 2001, 208). So what should most stand out in this context is the clear articulation of the idea that sad stories elicit negative emotions in the listener. Her story could really make me sad. And indeed, many people indicated that one must be sensitive to the effects of one's own speech on the emotions and reactions of others. Emotions, in lay terms, are construed as contagious—and the expression of negativity is understood to have ill effects for both the giver (who resubstantiates transient negative states in the telling) and the receiver (who is subject to share them). In turn, it is best to refrain from such dynamics for the psychological (and karmic) well-being of all.

Julia Cassaniti interrogates similar patterns of psychosocial support in her 2015 book, *Living Buddhism: Mind, Self, and Emotion in a Thai Community*. Her ethnography is filled with examples of displacement of emotional drama and the maintenance of "cool hearts" (*jai yen*, ใจเย็น) in the face of tumult. Rather than presuming her friends squelch their "true" feelings to maintain social norms or aim to keep emotions inside, she found people striving not to keep emotions at all. She describes this as a "local psychological model of health and well-being" that involves "letting go of attachments as part of a broader system of cause and effect" (Cassaniti 2015, 177 and 158). Calmness, Cassaniti attests, is a "moralized affective orientation" to the world (31).[10] The moral overtones stem from the karmic framework. Calmness is beneficial: both an ideal and an effect of merit-making.

My work similarly affirms the importance of karma in relation to these psychological dynamics. I also agree with Cassaniti that "it is both the symbolism of the action and the action itself that make the merit" in ritual activities (Cassaniti 2015, 98). But in marking the relationship between affect and effect, Cassaniti highlights the general folk correlation between good intention and good karmic outcome. Indeed, people explicitly affirmed the link between intention and merit in Cassaniti's interviews. When asked, interviewees would stress how "acting with good intention leads to good results, and acting with bad intention produces bad results" (160). But *how* they expressed this link may be telling. Making merit "in a huff" or a "bad mood" is considered unbeneficial; to illustrate, one man "[mimicked] pushing something toward someone gruffly, with eyes averted" (98–99). In turn, one might extrapolate how good manners and a placid exterior are just as crucial for these practices. In addition to self-reporting, what is emphasized or taught regarding merit-making activities is instructive; to that end, I found it is precisely external behaviors and appropriate preparation of offerings, rather than internal orientations, that are stressed as beneficial in merit-making.

I do not disagree entirely with this general association of good intention and good outcome. I do, however, think Cassaniti provides one additional clue that warrants further discussion of this correlation: "Actions done without intentionality do not create karma" (Cassaniti 2015, 159). I want to suggest that the mere possibility of an absence or neutrality of intention, which evades karmic accrual, is crucial for understanding the larger Buddhist soteriological project and its associated theory of mind.[11] This in turn can bring forth a fuller sense of the affective valence of caregiving in particular, and psychosocial support more generally, in northern Thai contexts. So in order to understand the karmic importance of intention and gain greater clarity on the parameters of this logic overall, I turn now to a Theravada (or Abhidhammic) theory of mind.

An Abhidhammic Theory of Mind

The Tipitaka—the compendium of sermons, commentaries, and technical manuals of the Theravada Pali Canon—is a productive resource for exploring alternatives to the dominant Western psychological theory of mind. Pali scholar

Maria Heim's 2014 book, *The Forerunner of All Things: Buddhaghosa on Mind, Intention, and Agency*, provides access to these texts in a holistic manner previously unavailable in the English language. Using Buddhaghosa's fifth-century commentaries as a guide, Heim unearths a sense of the philosophy's phenomenological and therapeutic implications, with each genre of the Canon providing a different angle from which to understand the whole. To my reading, she offers access to a key frame of reference beyond reported dogma—a mode not only of understanding the world, but also of engaging with it.

The third "basket" of the Canon, the Abhidhamma, is of a particular interest, as it presents a robust understanding of mind in technical detail.[12] The basic components of mind are identified in the Abhidhamma as individuated entities that are bundled together in any given instance to constitute experience. The mind's composition is both active and passive, with past actions determining which combinations or "choices" are possible in any given instance. Heim invites us to appreciate the play of possibilities evident here. That factors, or *dhammas*, appear across lists and in reference to different phenomena reflects the inexhaustible combinations possible depending on the particular circumstance.[13] Conditioning is essential to human experience and action; even perceptions themselves—what people can and do perceive through their senses—are in part a function of karma. For those who are able, karma is discernable as operating across lifetimes; for others, acknowledgment of the general process suffices.

Intention, or *cetanā*, in this lineage is an ever-present component of experience—but again, it is but one of many factors that make up the mind. As Heim explains,

> That intention belongs to the first five prereflective factors of consciousness, universally present in every conscious moment, means that intentions are always present in conscious experience. Also, they themselves are not morally valenced; they become good, bad, or neutral depending on which other factors occur within a thought moment. We can also see that the presence of so many factors of mental life relevant for thought and action decenters *cetanā* from being an isolated or discrete mental state that is solely responsible for the moral quality of karma. (2014, 102)

Experience is conditioned, made up by constituent parts that themselves are the consequence of karma across lifetimes. What's more, according to Heim, "our intentions can be influenced by others" through various forms of prompting (2014, 125). Present experience is therefore not independent of the past, or of the sway of others. And in this cycle of conditioning, every action—of body, speech, and mind, all of which have intention among their bundled component parts— is said to beget more karma; every action, that is, except for those composed of factors that do not bear karmic fruit, the *kiriya*. As discussed above, acting with no intention maps onto the *kiriya* of "fruitless intention"—neither bearing nor begetting karma.[14]

The absence of intention in this sense—action that does not produce karma—is beyond the reach of most ordinary people.[15] Intention-less action and non-karmic acts are the purview of *arhats* and the Buddha. Buddhist soteriology describes a path (the Noble Eightfold Path) to the cessation of karma and human suffering, though in the Theravada lineage its attainment is expected to take lifetimes. The awareness of suffering, its cessation, and the path to its cessation indeed involve a series of factors, from "right view" and "right action" to "right concentration," but intention itself is not the site of moral cultivation. The teachings point instead to restraint and discipline. Rather than technologies for developing positive attributes, Heim highlights the focus on *absence*. That is, positive traits are defined mainly as the absence of the negative.[16] One should refrain from a series of "bad" entanglements in the development of ethical sensitivity and the leading of a moral life en route to liberation. As Heim goes to great pains to show, "The path to *nibbanā* is *not* paved with good intentions" (2014, 61); rather, it is most readily promoted through restraint and discipline.

Restraint, rather than positive intention, is the key means by which people can properly condition their experience. After all, intention itself is subject to conditioning. As Heim puts it, "The basic logic is that it is only through restraint of the senses and of bodily and verbal action that the religious life can be lived and joy can be found" (2014, 140). This does not imply a sinning nature to be tamed. Unlike the Christian hermeneutics of ferreting out assumed impurity, refraining in ways prescribed by the Pali Canon allows for the spontaneous enactment of the good. Following dictums—such as the disciplines laid out in the Vinaya (the moral code of conduct for aesthetics), the five precepts for lay practitioners, and so forth—"'leads to restraint, restraint leads to nonremorse, nonremorse leads to joy, joy leads to delight, delight leads to calm, calm to happiness,' and so on all the way to *nibbana*" (Heim 2014, 138). The soteriological process is set on subjective experience, but indirectly: acceptance of "patiency" (as Heim calls the passive nature of moral action) and abstinence from harmful acts of body, speech, and mind create the conditions of attainment in the mundane practices and allegiances formed as a result.

It is my contention that the restraint prescribed in the canonical texts maintains great relevance for the sharing of emotions in the social world to this day. Such restraint is based on a theory of mind in which intention is karmically and interpersonally conditioned. Everyone in Thailand may not explicitly articulate this theory of mind, but it is regularly implied in common sense and embodied in ordinary practice. On one hand, one is subject to a constant flux of influences, internal and external, along a karmic time continuum. On the other hand, people talk and behave as if these influences should not upset one's mental state. Here lies the heart of ethical obligation. One should strive for—and the social world should support—actions and affects that minimize increases in karmic burdens. Karmic results, habit, and the influence of others are here incorporated in a complex model of interdependent intersubjectivity. The power of social values of equanimity and aesthetic appeal stems from this: at root, such states are conducive for the alleviation of karma, individually and collectively, on the road to liberation from suffering.

People I spoke to used a variety of metaphors that conveyed a sense of the hazardous nature of tumultuous states. For instance, one village eldercare volunteer described the danger in terms of a flood. She said that people generally do not want to "open their heart" because "a flood" could ensue—a flood of negative emotions that would overtake one's life and that of others as well. She certainly hinted to me over the course of our interactions that she knew about such potential, given her role as the main caregiver in her family, for her elderly mother as well as for her two brothers, who had died, respectively, of AIDS and alcoholism. Yet she kept a tight rein on her descriptions of these events, indicating pain without divulging details of her inner states. This woman's conduct and self-reporting represent, as clearly as common Jataka stories, the way emotions are understood as "contagious," and just how vulnerable ordinary people can be.

What's more, internal states are subjective clues to the state of one's karmic accrual. Negative sensations and emotional tumultuousness co-arise with "bad" actions. And, as Jidtuporn told me, one's inner state is a result of past karma as well. With upset an indication of negative karma, the best course of action is to downplay its arising and carry on according to social norms of comportment. This is understood in a variety of ways. Another friend, a masseuse named Mam, shared with me her philosophy regarding her role as a de facto consultant/adviser to her clients and friends. Mam stressed that she does not ask too many questions because that would only lead people to think more and make their lives miserable. Instead, Mam often challenges people by asking, "What if you died tomorrow and you were angry and stressed today? . . . You would," she says, "be heartbroken." What a waste of a short life!

Common narratives also make abundantly clear that although emotions can drive action, such feelings have complicated backstories. The Buddha or other enlightened beings can draw attention to past lives, which can clarify the source of present conflicts. For instance, there is a popular Jataka story (with many versions) in which a woman beats a group of monks after the loss of her husband. By showing the relationship between the monks and the woman across time, one can see beyond the present circumstances to the forces compelling their behavior. And indeed, many people to this day seek out guidance from trusted advisers regarding the seeds of their current affairs.[17] Rather than delving into the emotional states, "the real moral work here is properly framing the action" (Heim 2014, 194)—in particular, drawing attention away from the immediate emotional substrates to previous conditioning in a larger temporal sense.

So again, it is not that people never voice their emotional turmoil, but that framing or reframing it en route to equanimity is of utmost importance. Mam does this work, too. For example, she related to me a horrifying story about talking her friend out of murder. One night this friend had called her husband, who inadvertently answered his cell phone, allowing her to listen to him having sex with another woman. She was frantic when she talked with Mam, recalling in fury every detail of the forty minutes she had spent listening to the act of infidelity. She had clearly not "held it in" in some heroic philosophical act of reticence. The story came pouring out to a trusted confidante, who listened and reasoned with her not to kill her husband, despite his treacherous behavior. For Mam, this story reiterated not the benefit of emotional sharing, but rather the importance of refraining from fanning the flames of internal fire. There must certainly be karmic roots to misfortune. What of the consequences of following the path of retribution? There are of course times like these when direct engagement is necessary, but the goal for Mam is always to help others escape the cycle of negative thinking (and resultant negative emotions and negative actions) as soon as possible.

Heim's rendering of ancient Theravada thought allows us to appreciate how centuries-old ideas play out in the contemporary social world, just as they appear in different registers across the "three baskets" of the Pali Canon. Whereas, for instance, the Abhidhamma speaks with precision about the component parts of consciousness, the Suttas use the simple gloss of thinking and mind interchangeably (see Heim 2014, 134).[18] This is not because the Suttas are dumbed down; rather, the focus and audience is different, and what can be parsed in this other way of speaking is simply another avenue of exploration. Similarly, stories, which form such a considerable portion of Theravada literature, bring new appreciation to the more technical renderings of human experience found elsewhere. The link I want to make is this: Heim shows a new way to read Pali literature, seeing how the teachings cross-reference and build on one another in different registers across different forms of texts and commentaries. So, too, one can begin to see how the register of contemporary social interaction correlates with, plays out, and expands this base literature. Some speak fluently in dharmic language, while others deploy gross terms in seemingly contradictory ways—just as certain manual texts use precise technical terminology, and other texts present narrative depictions of dharmic logic in social context. And just as any given American may not, for instance, refer directly to Kant but may still hold and propagate a derivative notion of freedom and individual ethical choice, we can begin to trace a lineage of common sense in Thailand from figures in this tradition.[19]

In these philosophical underpinnings, we can see that emotion is a marker for and means of religious attainment. A "don't ask, don't tell" logic of intra- and interpersonal support thus reflects Theravada soteriology. *Jai yen*, or a cool heart, is associated with an acknowledgment of karmic conditioning and provides a calmness that is supportive (or otherwise indicative) of a break with worldly attachments. Through tempered emotional displays one can also find an acknowledgment of the complex workings of intersubjectivity, in which "emotions" are contagious attributes of mind spreading interpersonally and can be real impediments to the discipline of the Buddhist path. Where Cassaniti goes to a Western glossing of affect to make sense of "the high value placed on low arousal in the idiom of the cool heart" in Northern Thailand (see Cassaniti 2015, 81–82), I argue we can and must look to "indigenous" theories of mind for a more robust theoretical framework. Indeed, it is here that we can be awestruck at the continuities in the Theravada tradition—even in the midst of a range of other influences in the contemporary social world.

Sriwan's Story

I first met Sriwan in November 2008. She was spending most of her time alone on the steamy second floor of her wooden house in Chiang Mai city, lying in bed with an electric fan pointed at her chest. Her hair was dark and short, and despite being bedridden, she looked considerably younger than her eighty years. It was relatively cool outside, given the time of year, but the room was stuffy and warm, and the dark walls and lack of natural light intensified the depressed mood of the small place.

Sriwan was in enormous pain. She found it excruciating to walk and often painful just lying down motionless. She was deeply troubled, recounting her last several visits to doctors who could tell her nothing about her condition. She feared a return of the cancer she had fought nearly ten years before, but there was no word yet to that effect. With no medical explanation, she turned to a psychic, who traced the cause of her pain to a wandering spirit, the angry ghost of a young man killed at a nearby intersection. She had followed the psychic's advice, making merit for the spirit at a nearby temple and placing flowers and incense at the intersection itself, all to no avail. She was left wondering about the state of her karmic burden and fearing the unknown. All she wanted to talk about was the uncertainty; all she wanted, it seemed to me at the time, was to *know* what was ailing her.

Flash forward to August 2009. After many months of in-patient treatment at a hospital near Bangkok, Sriwan was back in Chiang Mai. I first heard she was back from a friend of hers, who told me she was in the terminal phase of bone cancer. Now she lay in a bed placed in the airy and open first floor of her daughter's home. Neighbors came and went at ease, able to call to her from the street and pop in without entering the private reaches of the house. Her hair was now completely white, looser and longer than I had seen it before. Twice a week her daughter or her daughter-in-law would place a plastic sheet on her bed and wash her hair for her. She was catheterized and completely dependent on these two women, who washed and changed her daily, prepared her meals, adjusted her TV and radio, brought her Buddhist sermons on tape, and sat to chat briefly throughout the day. Her two-year-old granddaughter too would come and amuse her, drawing pictures and romping around her queen-sized bed.

The environment stood in stark contrast to that of her old room; it was not only bright and light, but jovial. What had changed? Had she finally gotten clarity about her medical situation? Was she peacefully approaching an expected death? Not exactly. Before I visited, I was told I must be careful not to say anything about her bone cancer. Her old friends, her children, her husband, her neighbors, everyone knew she had this bone cancer—everyone, that is, except her.

I was not exactly surprised. Thai families often do not share a prognosis with a patient.[20] I had heard many times how sharing such news could, and regularly did, hasten the death of a person. Sriwan was a case seemingly in point—the doctors had told her family she would be dead by June, yet here she was months later in the foyer, conversing with all who cared to visit.

Over the course of several visits, I did find it remarkable that Sriwan was no longer focused on gaining specific certainty on her condition. She told me about her time in Bangkok, but only in brief; flanked as we were by family members, I felt a slight tension, like hackles rising, whenever our conversation ventured too close to treatment of her physical state. Instead, we focused on her experience as a volunteer in the past, and I dutifully interviewed her in this semipublic space in a way that allowed her to relive certain memories and share her former exploits. But away from her bedside, as I helped prepare food and readied the table with the family, we would sometimes whisper about her diagnosis—and it was only in these hushed encounters that I gleaned a few details of her case.

Then one day I happened to sit alone with the old woman, the rest of the family busy with other chores. We began to talk about her illness. She was relating details of her time in Bangkok, but abruptly stopped her description when she saw, out of the corner of her eye, her daughter approaching. As I recounted in my field notes:

> She gets a kind of wild look in her eye when talking about her illness now. Before it was a litany of despair; now, it's like sneaking to describe what

has been said and what she has gleaned, stopping when her daughter is near. . . . I wonder if she is searching my face for clues, I wonder if she wonders why I don't ask more directly or more often what the doctors have told her, etc.

One might wonder if my presence as an ethnographer and my former line of questioning provoked this encounter. Or one might wonder exactly how much she "knew" of her condition. There she was, surrounded by those dearest to her—her husband, her children, her closest friend since elementary school. She had presumably spent a lifetime assessing their needs and supporting them in times of trouble. Could she read on their faces the secret they shared about her?

Thinking "abhidhammically" about this situation alters such questions. Neither the "truth" of a diagnosis nor the space to discuss the emotional contours of approaching death has the greatest moral import in a Theravada frame. Karmic seeds span lifetimes to bear the fruit of a terminal cancer. Prognostic metrics are but one way of measuring such developments. A human life presents the opportunity for making merit, for sowing seeds of "good" karma of thought, speech, and deed—or better yet, extinguishing such seeds altogether. Good support comes from positive influence, whether in dharma talks or light-hearted topics of conversation, anything that can ease her mind as they help restrain her speech and comfort her body. Indeed, I may create an alternative set of coordinates, but that too will be fleeting. Ultimately, Sriwan supports her family by allowing them to support her in this manner, as they all participate in the prevailing logic of don't ask, don't tell.

The philosophical system of the Pali Canon, as extolled by Buddhaghosa and rendered anew by Maria Heim, provides a theoretical framework with which to appreciate this ordinary logic. The rendering matters. Heim carefully documents how many modern interpretations of Buddhist texts have inadvertently distorted key concepts. Heim argues, for instance, that modern scholars (including Keown, Gombrich, Payutto) tend to interpret *cetanā* through a lens of rational choice.[21] She calls such moves a "grafting" of Western thought onto Buddhist thought.[22] Indeed, the danger of presuming the configuration and moral valence of component parts of experience emerges here for study of intention and care alike.

Anthropologists generally understand that models of the self and the mind differ across cultures; this Theravada lineage of thought allows for a rich examination of contrasts and the implications of such contrasts for other topics of investigation, including care. Heim, for example, draws attention to common assertions of the will and an internal conscience as essential to moral knowledge and guidance, along with "romantic, rationalist, and psychological conceptions of the self developed in modernity" (2014, 24).[23] Tellingly, she simply does not find parallels in the Pali sources she surveys. Intention is not simply a correlate of the Western notion of the will, guided or not by the moral barometer of the conscience. Intention instead is decentered in the Theravada tradition, one of many component parts of any given action, with important antecedents both active and passive. Just as analysis should not inadvertently sneak notions of a conscience into moral deliberation in Pali discourse, so too must it avoid centering psychological correlates in the logic of care. Even with affective orientations of key concern, I am showing how the mode of achieving such states is not through direct means. Portraying intra- and interpersonal care based on an understanding of the mind as individuated, agentive in isolation, or in concert with so-called hydraulic modes of therapeutic disclosure would do an injustice to the sophistication with which people orient to the world and provide for others in many Northern Thai contexts.

Disclosure and Authenticity

I walk into the session a bit late. It is the fall of 2008, and I am attending one of the increasingly prevalent end-of-life care trainings at a large teaching hospital in Bangkok. I am the only non-Thai, out of hundreds in attendance. Nevertheless, many of the breakout sessions and panels at this two-day event are titled in English, as is the conference itself ("Empowering Palliative Care Team"). Indeed, one could argue a major Western influence in palliative care in the Thai context, with connections to the international hospice movement. But this particular session stands out, as it is named, in Thai, *kāndūlǣ sangkhom* (การดูแลสังคม), which translates as "social caregiving" or, more directly, "taking care of society."

It is a classroom setup, and I enter in the middle of a series of exercises. We are instructed to write and draw answers to various questions, some quite probing, such as what we want at our funeral, and so forth. There are three organizers, all female: a petite professional woman, around forty years old, is in the lead, flanked by two younger NGO-activist types. They lead confidently. We, in turn, seem to follow their instructions.

We are then told to write a letter to a loved one who has died. The main organizer, who I will come to know as a Thai social worker named Bee, strikes me as a little ridiculous as she repeatedly picks up the tissue box, demonstrating her readiness to hand out tissues. As I look around, I certainly do not see tearful emotions registering on the faces around me; at that point, I had rarely seen public displays of that type in Thailand since beginning work there in 1999.

Then Bee stands at the front of the room and, in a sweet, lispy voice, asks for volunteers to share what they have written. A bit of uncomfortable laughter ensues, followed by an uncomfortable silence. Clearly there will be no volunteers outright. Waiting only a few seconds, Bee calmly pulls out the roster sheet from the breakout session. There are fifty of us in the room, all registered with coupons to participate. And that is it. She picks a name, calls it out, and the woman called has to step to the front of the room.

After a couple of quick presentations that miss the mark (sharing about other exercises concerning funeral ideas and so forth), Bee continues with the roster and reminds people to share their letters. The next "volunteer" begins by saying to whom her letter is addressed, and then starts to read. Her nervous laughter is met by the social worker, standing quite close, with a firm yet gentle touch on the arm. As her emotional outpouring intensifies, Bee wraps her hand around the woman's waist. Encouragement. The cracking of her voice, the verge of tears. Polite applause. And another name is called.

Next up, a woman slightly shaking. She is angling to skip her turn. She begins and then says she cannot go on. But Bee is giving her no option. She cannot sit down, as if they have agreed beforehand that this is important work and they will not let each other quit. The letter-reader cannot face the crowd. She turns around. With the social worker's arm firmly around her waist, and tissues taken up, she chokes through her entire letter. Warm applause. She takes her seat. And this goes on, several more times: tearful letters read with one's back to the crowd. And then it is over. A few words in conclusion, and everyone presses their palms together in a courtesy *wai* and politely files out.

The disclosure in this scene might seem to fit a logic of "*do* ask, *do* tell," more than its inverse. What's more, the promptness and intensity of emotion evoked in this session could lead us to think that common patterns of social conformity require a "holding" of emotions inside.[24] But I want to argue that we need not take these displays as proof of a hidden storm of emotions lurking beneath the surface throughout social encounters and personal exchanges. Nor need we presume these disclosures purport to unveil a hidden self. Paying close attention to the protocols deployed in this conference setting—the display of tissues, the coaxing of emotional displays—it could just as well be that participants caught on to the form and enacted what the organizers advised, more or less creating and amplifying particular emotional contours.

Here I explore a set of Thai initiatives aimed at training people to break the news of a terminal medical prognosis and make advanced directives. From one vantage point, we could see these initiatives deploying technologies of the self new to this context that involve confessional practices, with the cultivation of conditions in which people confess inner emotional turmoil and probe one another for authentic disclosure. But from another vantage, the self in question can be understood as continually reconstituted in relation to a collective rather than through individuated or otherwise autonomous striving, based in the theory of mind outlined above, in which one's intention, subjective experience, and even karmic accrual is fundamentally subject to the influence of others. From the latter angle, these workshops and their emotional displays line up with what McDaniel (2008) calls the "living episteme" of the Thai Theravada religious and social tradition. The techniques discussed, which fit in one way so squarely in a confessional frame, may also be creative pedagogies for the establishment of new forms that stem from received wisdom based on a Theravada theory of mind. And while fully immersed in contemporary conditions, external form may continue to trump any particular internal orientation to the disclosures involved.

Calibration

As she tells it, Bee had wanted to be a social worker since the age of ten. She describes going to an orphanage for blind children on a class trip and coming away with a profound sense of wanting to work for others. Now, decades later, she attributes her lack of burnout in part to her personal drive to be in the profession.

Bee is active with HIV/AIDS patients nearing the end of life and is a key player in the burgeoning palliative care movement. But since this movement is relatively new in Thailand, and Bee's career is already quite long, I asked her how she used to approach death with such patients. She told me that everyone used to be afraid—not of catching HIV, but afraid that their patients would die brokenhearted. "So we didn't talk to them about death at all. If they were really close to dying, we wouldn't visit them."

It was a dream that started to change Bee's attitude toward the dying. She told me about a patient, a man she had been close with over the course of his treatment, whom she had not seen before he died. They had had an argument that stained their relationship, and when he was back as an in-patient at the end of his life, she avoided visiting him: a combination of hard feelings, fear of provoking sadness, and discomfort with such situations in general. Just before his funeral, he came to her in a dream. He was healthy, though he appeared in a coffin. He said to her, "In Thailand, we cremate the body. Help lower me into the coffin." Helping to put a dead body in the coffin is a way of making merit. Bee interpreted the dream to mean him asking forgiveness, offering her a way of making merit so they could both cleanse the ill effects of their prior argument. But more than that, the dream affected her understanding of the needs of patients before their death. The dream had occurred ten years prior to our conversation, right at the start of palliative care beginnings in Thailand; shortly thereafter, when she was invited to start working on palliative care, she took the opportunity.[25]

Bee has an impressive ability—an imperative, really—to encourage people in emotional sharing. Listening to her assumptions about the boundaries of such solicitations reveals an understanding of mind quite different from, say, the Freudian unconscious or that which is portrayed by various hydraulic metaphors (like emotions that build up like water behind a dam until they are released), which circulate globally. For instance, one day she was telling me about a woman who was dying of cancer and the little boy she was leaving behind. Children are not allowed in the intensive care unit (ICU) in Thailand, unless a patient is about to die. So Bee sat with the little boy outside the ICU, preparing him for his final visit. She explained to him what he would encounter, what he would see, and coached him how he must not cry.

Knowing how essential emotional sharing was to her practice, I asked Bee why this was the case. Why must the boy not cry? She patiently explained that, in Buddhist beliefs, one must not cry around someone who is dying, for it will cause them to worry, and they will then be unable to pass to the next realm.

So here we have someone on the cutting edge, incorporating "modern" forms of palliative care, though calibrated to more traditional understandings of appropriate emotional sharing. The idea that hospital spaces, so similar in form around the world, would be governed by a different logic was intriguing to me. I pressed Bee further, asking if there were special rooms in the hospital that were appropriate for crying. Bee repeated my question back, nonplussed. She said, of course, there were spaces in front of every hospital building. These rooms were for many activities; for example, she said, one could go "support" (and here she used the English word), eat together with relatives, and so forth. So yes, there were rooms like that.

That I had never seen anyone cry in these usually open air, public spaces is made legible in the logic of don't ask, don't tell, per the Abhidhammic theory of mind. In public hospital spaces, one could go and be supported, though not by venting and crying. By eating together. By normal activities of interaction, meant to shift the focus of transient thoughts and emotions away from the unwholesome. Just as following the physical protocols of caregiving suffices to transform karma and merit, as explored in chapter 1, so the protocols of social interaction provide a framework for restraining the mind and speech from ultimately harmful or unhealthy engagements.

Structured Telling

A prime example of strategic attempts to change modes of communication near the end of life in Thailand comes in the form of a recurring workshop titled

Confronting Death Peacefully, run by a progressive Buddhist collective. These are intensive gatherings, with participants delving deeply into issues of death and dying over the course of a long weekend. Confronting Death Peacefully is in fact one of many of this type of workshop, on an array of topics, focused in one way or another on reflective practice or contemplative education. A consortium of groups is involved in these activities; this particular one, part of Phra Paisal's Phuthikā Network, focuses on death, dying, and volunteering.

The organizers used role-playing as a device to initiate the discussion of breaking the news of a terminal medical prognosis and making decisions about care options. I found these role-play experiences illuminating in terms of my own conditioning as well as the patterns I witnessed in those around me. While I can attest to only my own experience, I offer an ethnographic account of a role-play encounter to delve into more detail regarding habits of psychosocial support, old and new.

For the particular exercise in question, I was paired with a middle-aged nurse named Haley. She was affable but perhaps only half-heartedly engaged. She was attending the workshop with a group of colleagues from her hospital and was presumably there on work duty rather than of her own volition. So we teamed up, and then separated to get our respective roles. I was told that Haley, for this role-play, is a relative of mine. She is a driven woman, with an upper-management position at a growing company. As far as she knew, she was in for a routine treatment of a chronic condition and was eager to get back to work as soon as possible. But her family knew that in fact her condition had worsened: doctors had found an advanced stomach cancer and did not think she would make it out of the hospital this time at all.

As mentioned, Thai patients are regularly shielded from full knowledge of their diagnoses and prognoses, as is the case in other parts of Asia.[26] However, palliative and end-of-life care supporters—embracing global claims of holistic care that deal directly with people's hopes and fears surrounding their approaching death—have increasingly challenged this tradition. Readying the Thai populace for improved end-of-life care has led to much debate about the "right to know" one's diagnosis and to limited training for medical professionals about how to "break bad news."[27] This workshop, in part, can be understood as part of such efforts.

Here I was, cast as a relative of Haley, the dying patient with no knowledge of the extent of her physical ailments. I was brought in by her three daughters to help with the situation. These daughters, I was told, had been unable to get through to her, as she was completely focused on her work responsibilities, and they could not bring themselves to tell her the "truth" (truth here being the biomedical reality). So they had approached a trusted relative (me) to break the news.

This was not exactly a public performance—all participants were paired and found their spots around the conference hall to engage in the scenario among themselves. Only later would we come back together to reflect on the process. Haley knew only that she was stressed about work, in for a routine hospital check, and expecting a visit from a relative. I approached, pretending she was lying not on a conference room floor but atop a hospital bed. We greeted each other and proceeded in typical hospital visit fashion, at least at first. Had she eaten? Who had been to see her? How was she feeling? Soon the conversation turned to her work concerns. As I had been primed, I recognized her preoccupation with business and her eagerness to get back to her daily affairs. She admitted pain but remained steadfast in her conviction that her time in the hospital would be over in a few days.

The situation was intense and difficult. I felt I had to complete the goal of the role-play, so although it never felt exactly natural, I decided to push forward and talk frankly about what the doctors had told the family. But as the words left my mouth, I was struck with the uncertainty of prognosis in general and the subsequent strangeness of my act of "revelation." How could we all be so certain that this woman would not leave the hospital? Recalling work on the poor state of prognostic science, and the power of suggestion, the violence of my words hit me hard.[28] But I was unprepared for the strength of my partner's reaction. She completely refused to believe me. Anger and shock registered on her face, and I was left feeling powerless and tormented.

Later, all the pairs returned to the large group to review our role-plays. There, Haley confirmed the anger and shock she felt. She reflected that she would not believe such news coming from a layperson. Perhaps this was a function of her job as a nurse; whatever the reason, she was convinced that a medical professional necessarily had to be the one to break such news. Not everyone agreed. Many indicated that they had had a successful, emotional revelation. But for Haley, the role of the family was to give encouragement (*hai kamlang jai*, ให้กำลังใจ), or literally "heart power," not to discuss terminal prognoses and the prospects of death.[29] I discuss this type of encouragement below; for now, I simply mark the correlation between Haley's common sense in regard to the don't ask, don't tell logic of support. One follows norms of restraint for healthy support.

It is important to note that the participants were, on the whole, members of the middle class. They were, by and large, educated and urban, working either in the health-care profession or some cosmopolitan venture. But one woman stood out. June was "from the countryside." She was a heavyset woman who wore simple clothes and sat back a bit from the group. She was there with her daughter, a young physician researcher named Pat. Pat had attended the top university in the country on scholarship and now worked in Bangkok. She had invited her mother to attend the workshop to expose her to the mindfulness practices and contemplative gatherings that had become a fixture of Pat's own life—and, of course, to help her mother prepare for a peaceful death, whenever the time might come.

June took it all in stride. She was quiet in the large group discussions, but when we were sitting together at lunch she expressed her thoughts more freely. She shared that she had been brought into the "modern ways" (presumably by her daughter) and would thus want to know her diagnosis and prognosis. But as for her fellow villagers, she thought they would not. In her role-play, June approached the subject by telling her partner about another friend who had had the same condition. She did not, however, mention that this "other friend" had died. When I asked how the story would convey the news, she said simply, "Thai people would understand."

I did not have the opportunity to ask June's partner whether she had, in fact, understood the news from June's story. It is hard not to imagine that, if what people say is true, a typical Thai could read the expressions on a close friend's face and in their body language to understand grave concern. And although, relying on Western paradigms, we might presume such "mind reading" through intuition and presumption must certainly lead to miscommunications, we must also recognize that the exact "facts" are not exactly what is at stake. If we take seriously the Abhidhammic theory of mind and the Buddhist soteriological path to which it relates, a type of non-arousal is of vital importance. There is nothing to move through; as Mam related, what if one dies amid a storm of tumult? What a waste of a precious human birth. Following the forms of received wisdom in body, speech, and mind is understood as a better route to escape the cycle of human suffering.

Nevertheless, modern medical advances have indeed altered the conditions in which many people die, in Thailand as elsewhere. Given hospital settings and the potential for deploying intensive technologies in the last days of life, aiding low arousal may require new strategies. Contemplating potential scenarios, such as those facilitated by these workshops, deploys forms familiar to Western contexts but perhaps with an alternate telos. To consider this possibility, I delve further into fundamental coordinates of lived experience.

Kamlang Jai: The Experience of Encouragement

When asked what one should do when visiting a sick person, an old person, a person close to death, the answer people provide is nearly always the same across Thailand: give them encouragement, or *hai kamlang jai* (ให้กำลังใจ).[30] Although it is difficult to pin down exactly what is involved in that action, giving "heart power" is often thought to involve shielding weak patients from hearing news that could shock them into an early demise. Instead, one must focus on the positive, tell them they are doing well, fulfill their desires, maybe give them a case of Brand's (แบรนด์) drink, and keep their environment free from stress and strain.

Venturing to describe what it is like to experience *kamlang jai* is a daunting task. But I can relate one window I had into such a state, again from a role-play situation at this same workshop. In this scenario, I was given the role of a patient in a hospital. I was feeling horrible and could sense my condition was worsening. What's more, I was far from serene. All my worries and anxieties were focused on my two children, ages eight and twelve. I was concerned about their future, about who could care for them. Their father had to work long hours in a province far away, and I feared they would be abandoned. To prepare for my role, I mimicked the physical stance I had witnessed in others close to death. I conjured up the physical exhaustion I myself have experienced in times of sickness, and I let my mind go off into worst-case scenarios about the lives of two children without a mother to care for them.

In came my partner. Her bright and cheery attitude was immediately off-putting to me, a bolt of energy completely antithetical to the internal experience I had cultivated. Although I answered her initial questions about my eating and my visitors, I felt my own expectations rise in a cloud of anger and confusion at what felt to me like a superficial conversation. I pushed forward to confide my anxieties about my kids. She was overly eager to soothe in response. She did not seem to register my criticism that her words and demeanor were too fast, too much, and that all I wanted was a good listener. I found myself crying.

Her motions were fast. She was consoling and placating, but I did not find this comforting. Was this *kamlang jai*? She said things like, "Don't worry, your mom can take care of your children." She was smiling a lot. Touching my hands. I was completely overwhelmed.

At some point, I began to feel that I had better tell her it was okay, so that she would not feel bad, so that she would not think her actions were in vain, so that somehow we could amicably conclude the visit. I forced a smile; I told her she was right.

Remarkably, in that way, I did, in fact, begin to feel better. Was this the cycle of *kamlang jai*? A "fake it until you make it" social norm? Regardless of whether my personal experience—contrived as it was—can compare with that of a patient on their deathbed, it does resonate with forms of mutual support that I witnessed between caregivers and care-receivers. Take Sriwan, the woman living out her days in her daughter's home, with everyone around her shielding her from her diagnosis. Questions of how much she "knew" about her condition detract from an appreciation of the dynamic played out between her and her relations as they kept up appearances. Engaged in light conversation with a neighbor, having her hair washed, or even listening to the array of religious tapes made available to her within arm's reach of her bed—these are a stockpile of "positive" inputs. Her pain was well managed with medications, and the taped sermons were in large part instructions for dealing with physical discomfort. Even if I did catch a glimpse of some eagerness to discuss her medical condition, the Theravada theory of mind and the transience of thoughts therein would not have us assume this was an ever-present desire waiting for the right person to come by to relieve it.

June seemed to practice *kamlang jai* in her countryside style, too. She considered using coded language—telling a dying woman a story about another person in a similar situation, rather than directly recounting a terminal diagnosis—as an appropriate approach to supporting someone at the end of life. But while it may be possible that people are so practiced in telegraphing needs and assessing the desires of others that such an example might create the conditions for understanding, new medical technologies create unfamiliar conditions that may no longer allow old forms of symbolic communication to suffice. But what needs to change is up for debate.

Social scientists have studied how new technologies create new communication needs the world over.[31] Again, part of the intention of the workshops and trainings described above is to change people's communication style in the face of medical advances.[32] Now, although these groups seem to facilitate new conditions that defy the logic of psychosocial support I have claimed above, they are nonetheless relying on old social patterns that are part and parcel of that logic. For instance, although the Confronting Death Peacefully workshop may have similarities with any number of self-help-type workshops in the United States, it takes place in a setting where participants have been brought up to intuit what is expected and to provide accordingly. I am arguing that we cannot read these spaces as simply a rare opportunity for people to share their "true" inner emotional states.[33] Such a move not only delegitimizes widespread strategies of encouragement, intimacy, and psychosocial support; it also serves to cast out the entire theory of mind as irrelevant and replace it with something more akin to a hidden unconscious or otherwise independent notion of the self. I find it more compelling to read these initiatives as an attempt—a successful one, at least in the moment, for the majority of participants—to create a space for a particular form of sharing and reflection. This pivots on expectations created within the group about what is desired by group facilitators, what constitutes "fitting in" in this particular setting, and so forth.[34] Confronting Death Peacefully and other training programs seem to offer direct emotional sharing as a means of support, though "authentic disclosure" may be less at stake than creating new social forms that assist with old patterns of replacement and restraint.

New Forms, Old Forms:
Moral Life in the Thick of Things

In the introduction to his new translation of the *Therigatha*, a collection of poems by the first Buddhist women, Charles Hallisey draws attention to a poem by Chanda.[35] As he assesses it, "It is clear that she decides to ordain as a Buddhist nun not out of any spiritual aspiration but as a way of getting food" (Hallisey 2015, xxx).

> In the past, I was poor, a widow, without children,
> without friends or relatives, I did not get food or clothing.
>
> Taking a bowl and stick, I went begging from family to family,
> I wandered for seven years, tormented by cold and heat.
>
> Then I saw a nun as she was receiving food and drink.
> Approaching her, I said, "Make me go forth to homelessness."
>
> And she was sympathetic to me and Patachara made me go forth,
> she gave me advice and pointed me toward the highest goal.
>
> I listened to her words and I put into action her advice.
> That excellent woman's advice was not empty,
>
> I know the three things that most don't know,
> nothing fouls my heart.

The poem points to enlightenment ("I know the three things that most don't know, / nothing fouls my heart"), a state gestured toward but not fully explained, or explainable, to those who have yet to come to comprehend the teachings of the Buddha. But taking the advice of sages and following the dictates of tradition is essential. "I listened to her words and I put into action her advice." And it is going through the motions—for instance, shaving one's head and donning robes, in the case of an aesthetic—that leads to profound spiritual attainment. Here intentions are not emphasized. What motivates advised actions matters less than the habits to which one subjects oneself.

As argued in chapter 1, the power of one's action can be embedded in the physicality rather than in one's internal orientation. *I want food, I don robes, I become a stream non-enterer or achieve enlightenment*; likewise, *I change diapers, and whatever my motivation to the task, my karmic coordinates change*. A focus on bodily actions was necessary to unsettle dominant understandings of care, in which scholars imply a conscience-led internal orientation is critical to care. But thoughts and feelings are of course part of life as well. In light of the Abhidhammic theory of mind, we can refine this equation. The Abhidhamma provides a subtle rendering of component parts of experience, in which one's mind-states are highly relevant but conditioned: manipulable by external influence, physical actions, and forms of restraint more readily than from direct cultivation, but again, always karmically contingent. Thus, an important contrast between this Thai case study and the Christian hermeneutical tradition of self-reflection comes to the fore.

One way to understand this is through the genealogy of practices Foucault traces in his lectures in *Technologies of the Self*.[36] Early Christian practice centered on self-contemplation to ferret out hidden secrets, like lust; in turn, verbalization became essential to marking the truth in the form of confession. Anything that could not be verbalized was cast as sinful. Obedience went hand in glove with contemplation for early Christian monastics; thus renouncing oneself to one's master (as to God) lay at the heart of the confessional technologies Foucault outlines. But this practice shifted with time. According to Foucault, "From the eighteenth century to the present, techniques of verbalization have been reinserted in a different context by the so-called human sciences in order to use them without renunciation of the self but to constitute, positively, a new self" (1988, 49). Although the lack of renunciation constitutes a break in this lineage, there is nonetheless a continuity of self-care behaviors rooted in confessional technologies from Augustine through Freud.

Important differences remain between the practices of self-examination and disclosure in the Christian tradition that Foucault details and the patterns of practice in the Theravada Buddhist tradition as I gloss it here.[37] In particular, in the latter, there is not the emphasis on "deciphering . . . inner thoughts," with the implication of "something hidden in ourselves," as Foucault describes for both early Christian and modern liberal hermeneutics of the self (1988, 46). The focus remains on interiority and an alignment between inner thoughts and feelings (which require scrutiny for proper ascertainment) and outward actions. And although there is a kind of "obedience" to be found in following the advice of Buddhist sages, and a kind of "contemplation" to be unearthed in Theravadin aesthetic practices, the Abhidhammic theory of mind has alternate coordinates.

Buddhist temple rituals as well as rituals of care are successful in transforming merit through actions; little emphasis is placed on an agreement between inner orientation and external actions. Thus we must not demand such agreement in the reading of "good care" in such a context. Similarly, techniques for eliciting particular forms of internal reflection need not map onto "hidden" or otherwise preexisting constituents of personhood stifled by social structures. Although the don't ask, don't tell framework may be transformed through confessional technologies, an underlying notion of a transient self may persist. The solicitation of temporary states for communications deemed necessary in the contemporary context does not necessarily displace an underlying Abhidhammic theory of mind. In this way, what Heim calls "technologies of restraint" are harnessed and cultivated to influence the component parts of experience. Motivations and other aspects of thought may ultimately matter for the specific contours of karmic outcomes, but if emphasis in practice is any indication, they are most effectively manipulated indirectly.

Hallisey advocates an appreciation of moral life not from the standpoint of dramatic decision-making points, but rather from life in the thick of things. He thus points to the Theravada ethical value of enacting the sound advice of sages and the dictates of tradition as living the good life. In this chapter, I have attempted to excavate the roots of psychosocial behavior that fit such an ethical schema. A logic of don't ask, don't tell has propagated in Thai social worlds, whether attached to an explicitly Buddhist frame or not. I have attempted to elucidate the lived experience of these patterns of intra- and interpersonal support, along with the local theory of mind that supports them. As Veena Das writes, "Because of the strong emphasis on intentionality and agency in our contemplation of ethics, habitual actions are often reduced to 'mere behavior'" (2012, 139). This is as true in psychosocial realms as it is in physical domains. Indeed, the two are interrelated.

In chapter 3, I attend to habituated actions in the thick of group social interactions. I look closely at how perceptions are trained through repetition of social forms, naturalizing entrained assessments of the world. Social dictates order what stands out in the environment as most important, and thus becomes the world as perceived. Describing in detail what stands out in collective settings rounds out a preliminary picture of a generalized mode of being—from the embodied actions at bedsides, through forms of emotional parsing, to ways of perceiving as part of a group—that are foundational to the lived experience of caregiving. Attending to the process of providing for others, we can see more clearly dynamics of social change, in terms of both standard domains of care and care in the larger contexts of interpersonal and political action. Indeed, phenomenological training of awareness can serve at times to mask the effects of power through habituation to the social world; my analysis in this regard serves to outline the stakes of ordinary care in practice across various realms of the social world.

THE SUBJECTS OF CARE

Perceiving the Social Body

On the surface, the proceedings of professional conferences may appear fairly generic; whether staged in large banquet halls and auditoriums or in more intimate
conference rooms and classrooms, recognizable formats abound. Panelists take
their seats facing the audience, a speaker might stand at a podium, PowerPoint
slides might occasionally appear on a wall or a screen. Experts gather in these
spaces to share the latest information on the topic at hand, often with short presentations followed by questions or discussions among the group.

Despite their seeming universality, such events offer a fishbowl in which to
observe some of the rules of engagement particular to a given social group (see
Goffman 2005 [1967]). In a typical Thai context, an extra air of formality might
soon be detected. For instance, a certain exacting attention to detail might be
apparent, with speaker name cards neatly scripted and placed on starched
linen-covered tables, or a special area designated for VIPs to take their meals
(complete with ornately carved fruit or at least the choicest selection of dishes).[1]
One might notice how participants bow when entering or leaving the meeting
space. A scurry of young people might slide in and out of rooms, bent at the
waist so as never to rise above anyone's head, ensuring that all equipment is
functioning or that everyone important has water and knows the exact order of
events to come.

All these elements were apparent in February 2009 at a moderately sized, three-
day meeting on end-of-life care at a major hospital in Bangkok. Thai hospital
staff interested in or currently involved with palliative care efforts joined with doc-

tors, nurses, and social workers from Canada, all considered "experts" in end-of-life issues.

The event was arranged by a group of Thai nationals, all doctors, who had been living in the United States for decades. With Thailand seemingly frozen in time in their minds, these accomplished men wanted to "give back" to their homeland (raising their own status in Thai society in the process) by "bringing" palliative care to the Thais. Their vision was to create a "center for excellence" in palliative and end-of-life care that could become a model and a resource for the country at large. Hence the import of including leading North American figures, there to help set the stage and provide what was presumed to be the necessary training.

It struck me that nothing much had been communicated to this group about the decade-long palliative care movement already under way in Thailand or the center for excellence in end-of-life care already established in the southern province of Songkhla, or even the host institution's own experience with a long-standing palliative care service. But, in fact, the silence on this front was somehow not surprising. Thai experience with state-of-the-art palliative care would have been contradictory to the assumptions and intentions of the organizers. In this way, the overall conduct of the meeting speaks to the issues I raise in this chapter regarding social interactions. I intend to show how social norms cue a phenomenological training of awareness of utmost importance for the codes and conduct of care at a variety of levels, including care for one's group.

One incident in particular best introduces the contentions at hand. A well-known former monk and senior attendee, Dr. Itsara, was speaking to the Canadian panel about "Thai culture." He was highly educated and cosmopolitan, having spent a great deal of time abroad, and was at that time angling for either a government health minister position or a platform in the world of palliative care from which to launch his political aspirations. Speaking in impeccable English, he captured everyone's attention as he explained to the foreigners how crucial it was to understand that Thais have no concept of self-esteem. Therefore, to be effective, palliative care protocols would need to be tailored accordingly. The members of the panel were intrigued. Their eyes flashed with possibilities for cultural dialogue as they scribbled notes.

The panel was unaware, however, that sitting directly behind Dr. Itsara was a middle-aged female nurse who had in fact written her doctoral dissertation on the very concept of self-esteem that Dr. Itsara was claiming did not exist for Thais. Several people in the audience knew this, but no one raised a single point of contention, then or at any point in the proceedings thereafter. Later I asked this researcher what she thought of Dr. Itsara's comments. She admitted she thought many of his ideas were extreme, and said something about how people would not be able to work effectively if such notions were taken up in too radical a manner. But again, neither she nor anyone else openly disagreed or shared an alternative view during the conference.

The undercurrent in this story could be presented in many forms. What appears in such instances is a mode of indirectness and a glossing over of tensions for the maintenance of surface harmony, a way of behaving in public and semi-private arenas that de-emphasizes the individual as such and continually reinscribes hierarchical positions between people. Scholars have grappled with such aspects of Thai social relations for decades. Some have attempted to make sense of these social characteristics in terms of "face" and related concepts.[2] Yet even in the most rigorous linguistic and sociological studies, the concept of "face" falls short, for it fails to bring attention to the lived experience of group dynamics and the perceptual coordinates of the values that such interpersonal dynamics reflect and sustain. If instead we consider the ways in which Thai social interactions involve active attention to and care of the "social body," a new realm of power-infused habituated patterns of action becomes apparent.

Perception is at the root of the issue in the discussion that follows, in which I provide a sense of how Thai subjects feel themselves to be part of a group (on large and small scales), as well as how social, religious, and political structures are embodied through habituated means of perceiving as part of the collective. I show how norms of social engagement prioritize what stands out in the environment, how interpersonal interactions are both felt and valued, and how certain patterns of etiquette template moral actions as well as ethical reflection. When one is habituated to perceive oneself as part of a group in the ways I describe, actions to provide for that group according to social dictates function as a form of care for others and as a form of self-care.

This aspect of Thai society and social relations carries great import for the way policy is created and implemented, as well as for the various ways social support is sought and governed at the community level. It works hand in glove with the logic of psychosocial support I describe in chapter 2 and has bearing on the functioning of volunteer programs I explore in chapter 4. Finally, it provides a framework for understanding the political unrest that has uprooted the country since as early as 2006, alerting us to what is at stake for elites as well as the poor in these struggles that have led to bloody protests on the streets of Bangkok and elsewhere, which I interrogate in chapter 5. To understand the changes afoot in an "aging" Thailand, one must take into consideration the social body and the care people show to it. Likewise, to adequately understand the care shown to individuals, as well as the systems developed to support such care, one must be clear on the types of actions that constitute care at the interpersonal level and at community and institutional levels as well.

The Social Body

Although the term "social body" is not new, here I seek to alter its common use. Lawrence Cohen, Mary Douglas, Terence Turner, Emily Martin, and Veena Das punctuate the long list of anthropologists and sociologists who have evoked the term. It has, for instance, been powerfully deployed to highlight the metaphoric and symbolic usage of the human body in societies, including as a natural symbol for relationships in the environment and society (Douglas 1970). Scheper-Hughes and Lock (1987) advocated for examination of "three bodies"—the individual body, the social body, and the body politic—representing "not only three separate and overlapping units of analysis, but also three different theoretical approaches and epistemologies: phenomenology (individual body, the lived self), structuralism and symbolism (the social body), and poststructuralism (the body politic)" (1987, 8). One could consider my use of the term social body as an amalgamation of these three. I deploy the social body first as an analytic metaphor (that is, one not ethnographically prevalent but analytically useful). It serves to draw attention to the phenomenological training of awareness, through symbolism and institutionally mediated power, within collectives. One can then begin to appreciate a mode of perception and the resultant lived experience of being part of a group. Critiques of previous uses of the social body—including its functionalist, static, authoritarian, and idealistic undertones—are well taken. I am aware of no other use of the social body that attempts, as I do here, to illuminate the habituation of human bodies via social dictates into patterns of perception that serve to naturalize people feeling themselves as part of a group, part of a larger social body.

My argument does not posit a singular Thai social body or adherence to a fixed set of norms without dynamism or conflict. Rather, I seek transitory instances that illuminate this type of patterning precisely because of the ultimate flexibility of such conditioning. While I bring some important representational components of bodies to the fore, my central goal in using the term is to keep expanding the bounds of phenomenological analysis to include interpersonal and collective interactions in the training of awareness.

In what follows, I conceive of the "social body" primarily as an actual living organism of which everyone is a part. This is not an ontological assertion; rather, it is a conceptual formulation to bring attention to perceptual patterning.[3] From such a perspective, "group harmony" and its maintenance hold key significance.[4] If, as a prelude, we consider that "health" is to the individual body what "group harmony" is to the social body, then the import of so-called social unity begins to present itself. All the organs must be functioning; all systems must be operative and working in an integrated fashion with all other parts. For example, the kidneys cannot be expected to do the work of the liver, cells cannot reproduce at too fast a rate, and so forth. But it is not enough to stay at the metaphorical level with such terms, for it is in the momentary maneuvers and perceptual patterns performed and lived by members of groups that we can trace the significance of the "social body" as a conceptual tool. Thai social bodies, generally speaking, comprise various parts, all of which have their place based on the rules of social hierarchy.[5] Only certain individuals can act as the face of that body, directing its movement, at any given time. Committing attention to this collective requires the active surmising of these various roles and of one's own place in the group, a set of perceptions engaged whenever multiple people are gathered together; the "care" of this body then occurs in the maintenance of harmonious relations and the proper following of whoever is in the lead at any given moment (regardless of what may happen at a future point in time). In this way, people value and protect social unity alongside personal physical health and equanimity.

An increasingly clear impetus is apparent, in the literature of moral anthropology, to gain a critical edge or a social practice orientation to the phenomenology of individual experience. Attempts to do this vary. Some scholars look to Bourdieu alongside Husserl and/or Merleau-Ponty to expand their philosophical underpinnings and political relevance. Others turn to Heidegger, Foucault, Schutz, or Nietzsche to explore political relations, historical patterns, and ontological possibilities within contemporary phenomenological anthropology.[6] In this discussion I follow, in part, the former thread. The idea of the social body takes on Bourdieu's notion of straddling different ways of knowing—symbolic and material, objectivist and subjectivist—as the term refers simultaneously to a metaphorical model and a mode of perception.

I am dealing here with a general field of public and semiprivate interactions in urban Thailand. A "field" in this sense is not a rigidly fixed structure, but its relations are continually reproduced through creative participation with historically constituted forms of power (Bourdieu and Wacquant 1992, 16). Thinking Abhidhammically, a field, as any phenomenon, comprises a particular combination of component parts, their bundling a function of conditioning. Habitus is likewise conceived as historically constituted, embodied, and maintained in individual bodies. My analysis of habitus will unearth Bourdieu and Wacquant's sense of "perception, appreciation, and action" reflected in bodily comportment and physical interactions. Concurrently, my analysis of class and hierarchy helps display the relative weight of elements in this field, and brings possible trajectories for change into sharper focus. Although redirecting perception and retraining body movements is possible and could certainly create new patterns, in this chapter I focus on a set of practices and scenarios that reflect common values and moral action.

In Northern Thailand, a certain spiritual aspect of bodies is known as the *khwan* (ขวัญ); it can be understood as the "life force" or "spirit" of individuals as well as of communities (such as in the term *khwanmɨang*, ขวัญเมือง, or the spirit of the city).[7] To be appropriate in this context, correspondence between a healthy body and a healthy society must account for both the physical and spiritual attributes of bodies. Such links then play into phenomenological sensibilities. There are ceremonies and rituals for "calling back" *khwan* into individual bodies as well as into ailing villages (Tanabe 1991, 187). Individuals may serve as the embodiment of *khwan* for collectives: the king, as *dhammaraj*, could, for example, be understood as the guiding spirit for the society as a whole.[8] One might also conceptualize local leaders taking on a similar role in smaller scales.[9] At both individual and collective levels, disturbances to internal equilibrium can lead to the flight of *khwan* and the loss of health or life. Karma (*kam*) and destiny (*chata*) are also potential threats to the internal equilibrium that defines good health, but anthropologist Shigeharu Tanabe asserts that, "compared with *kam* and *chata*, spirit [*khwan*] brings more direct and specified effects on the equilibrium to be sustained both in the soul body unity and social relations." Importantly, this is not merely a philosophical axiom but rather is central to daily existence. Tanabe argues, "The power of the spirit is, as [Benedict] Anderson suggested in the case of Java, not a theoretical and abstract postulate, but concrete existential reality" (1991, 187).[10]

The task at hand is to locate the perceptions that undergird these classifications, the manner of forming relationships between bodies perceived in these ways, and the values those relationships hold. The representational parameters of the body sketched above help make clear that, at the ideological level, harmonious equilibrium is essential to the conception of the health and well-being of individuals as well as collectives, and the body cannot be understood solely in physical terms.[11] How then do people sense (not just make sense of) the collectives in which they take part? And what analytical purchase might the "social body" bring to a discussion of Thai moral experience and the place of care therein?

Perceptions, Appreciations, and Actions

In a small meeting at a major research university in Bangkok, a group had gathered to plan the university-wide implementation of an innovative learning program. Key participants took their places at a long oval table, with several observers (myself included) seated off to the side. It was lunch hour, and boxed meals were served on trays with shiny silverware and napkins.

The university rector, Professor Prasert, arrived a bit late and took his seat at one end of the central table. At the other end sat Professor Apirak, a vice dean and the director of the program to be scaled up. These two professors were long-time colleagues and peers, though now that Professor Prasert was the rector, he was the most senior person present. Their status was marked when the food arrived. The attendants familiar with Apirak brought him lunch first; he bowed and insisted they serve Prasert before him; Prasert then deferred, in yet another demonstration of courtesy, claiming he was en route to another lunch meeting and would not be eating; and finally, the helpers retraced their steps to return the meal to Apirak. Third in rank was Professor Verde, a senior female faculty member. She had a great deal of management experience and would soon become an important player in the meeting. Others, younger or only distantly connected to the matters at hand, would play less prominent roles.

Prasert's role as the visionary, business-type leader was soon apparent, as he showered praise on Apirak's presentation and peppered his speech with abbreviations and catchphrases like "Think big but start small." Verde joined the discussion in an advisory capacity. Her comments reflected time spent in the United States, and she offered a Stanford University scheme as a possible model. Apirak maintained a measured presence, and once Prasert excused himself from the proceedings, Apirak took the helm as the undisputed leader of the meeting.

Soon after Prasert departed, something sparked a conflict. That is, something sparked a "Thai-style" conflict. The dispute arose so subtly that I missed the exact moment of disagreement. Suddenly, Prasert and Verde were locked in a barely perceptible argument—at least, barely perceptible to me—over strategy. They went back and forth, beginning their exchanges with courteous phrases to soften the blow of their words: a "Permit me to speak frankly" here, an "Excuse me" there. The sparring continued until Apirak was in fact interrupting Verde. And as Verde talked about competing time commitments, Apirak averted his gaze, with a hint of glaze coming over his eyes.

The tension was high, though you would miss it if you were looking for the sort of tension found in open disagreement, raised voices, or the thrown limbs of annoyance or disgust. Yet the discomfort registered around the room. People looked away, brushed crumbs from the table, cleared their plates. The woman next to me, another observer, was a case in point. As Apirak and Verde continued back and forth, she neatly packed her things and gathered her dishes, nearly quaking with uneasiness. In an exasperated voice, she whispered to me that she hated such an environment, and with that, she rose, quietly bowed, and rushed off.

It was not until someone else stepped in, another senior faculty member who had been silent through the proceedings, that the situation defused. He reminded everyone that this type of engagement would not make things better, and both parties gave him their attention in agreement. Eye contact resumed, and they made a plan for a three-day workshop in the near future to discuss the issue further. I later debriefed with this "peacemaker." He thought Verde was in fact playing the scapegoat for what was actually Apirak's anger toward his own staff for not doing more to help the program implementation get going. If such an interpretation is correct, the concept of "face" provides much traction for making sense of such a scene. The demure behavior of the combatants followed the rules of polite social interaction, and each worked actively to protect the "face" of the other, even as Verde more or less sacrificed her own face for Apirak's staff. But why were the other participants so visibly uncomfortable with the situation? Why was the woman next to me unable to bear witness to the exchange?

The Embodied "I"

If, as I am claiming, people can value cohesion in their groups just as they cherish the healthy functioning of their own bodies, how do they become attuned to that larger social body? As incarnated beings, it must at some level be a function of their own bodily processes. Merleau-Ponty argued for centrality of the body in this way, yet he also recognized that critical thought transcends direct worldly perception, "almost to the point of forgetting the contribution of perception to our idea of truth" (Merleau-Ponty 2004, 23). Somehow, we have to get a handle on how our bodily movements can be associated with, and perhaps even provide a window onto, both our immediate perceptions and our critical concepts. I find habit is one avenue for doing so, and I draw on continental phenomenology, together with contemporary cognitive science, to highlight a habituated link between culturally contingent values and sensory perception.

As Merleau-Ponty wrote, in *The Phenomenology of Perception*, "The acquisition of a habit is indeed the grasping of a significance, but it is the motor grasping of a motor significance" (Merleau-Ponty 2004, 164). The import of this statement is amplified by recent studies of functional neural systems, exemplified by the "enactive approach" of the late Francisco Varela. Varela sets his moves apart from the computationalist tradition in cognitive science, which understands the world as pre-given and therefore formulates cognition as an information-processing problem. Instead, echoing Merleau-Ponty, Varela asserts that we construct reality through our movements: what we touch, how we eat, as we breathe. Therefore, he argues, "The point of departure for understanding perception is the study of how the perceiver guides his actions in local situations" (Varela 1999, 12). What "counts" as relevant in the world depends on the perceiver. More precisely, it is one's movement through space that generates the differences that become observable, movement that allows figures to stand out against the ground, movement that generates meaningful perception. At root, I am arguing that the societal conditioning of habitual patterns—as constitutive of a field, as Bourdieu called it, and as embodied and reinforced via habitus—draws forth different modes of perceiving the world in general and, for the purposes of this chapter, distinct ways of sensing social relations in particular. Appropriate behavior in a meeting room, food delivery protocol, ways of entering and exiting a space, and other forms of etiquette are constituted in and by the body, and in turn they serve to naturalize assumptions about and assessments of the social world.

But it is not just individuals' perceptions of the group that are relevant; one must consider too the implied nature of bodies, individual and collective, as well. In particular, habits show that a central processing unit is not necessary for perceptual activity. Varela postulates that "cognitive structures *emerge* from recurrent patterns of sensory-motor activity" (Varela 1999, 16, emphasis original), underscoring that experience creates, reinforces, and confines neural pathways and thus creates, reinforces, and confines possibilities in understanding. Again, there is no central processing unit. Varela is talking about self-organizing systems with emergent properties: thus any "I" is, essentially, a virtual one. Varela thus claims that there are "*strong* metaphors, nay, exemplars, for what is a selfless self: a coherent whole that is nowhere to be found and *yet* can provide an occasion for the coordinated activity of neural ensembles" (1999, 60, emphasis original).[12] The social body, as I am deploying the term, is based in part on these metaphors: "The Selfless 'I' is a bridge between the corporeal body which is common to all beings with nervous systems and the social dynamics in which humans live" (Varela 1999, 62). People come to share and embody conventional understandings of being "I"s in the world, just as they share values, habits, and preferences.

Marking participation in the social body is akin to assessing this emergent and interdependent nature of existence. Of course, the Thai social world does provide well-worn pathways to central authority; groups accept leaders and their positions of authority, just as individuals come to naturalize their own sense of "I," even if, ultimately, those pathways are a result of simple repetition. In this way, all "structure" should be understood as constructed. It may be that recognizing the typified "structure" of the social body will allow for the identification of "structural violence," that is, harms imposed by these social forms. This, then, is a necessary first step in extricating the moral logic and the embodied dispositions that function to naturalize social rules. Discomfort registers around the room in response to a dispute among leadership, a disruption of habituated patterns in this local moral world.

Physical Coordinates

With the above cognitive foundation, Varela helps us see habitual actions—rather than conscious judgments and abstract assertions—as the spontaneous and embodied root of moral activity. Varela in this way inspires my rendering of habituated action as the heart of morality, as described in the introduction, as well as resonates with Maria Heim's recent call to look to "moral anthropology" to advance the study of Buddhist ethics and "the intersubjective nature of the human condition" (Heim 2011, 583). In particular, Heim urges analysis of "everyday activities of perception and attention" (583), which she claims can reveal a rich range of moral action that informs the formulation of, and rational deliberation about, ethical concerns in a given context. As Varela similarly describes,

> A wise (or a virtuous) person is *one who knows what is good and spontaneously does it.* It is this immediacy of perception and action which we want to examine critically. This approach stands in stark contrast to the usual way of investigating ethical behavior, which begins by analyzing the intentional content of an act and ends by evaluating the rationality of particular moral judgments. (Varela 1999, 4, emphasis original)

In essence, Varela is asking philosophers to take seriously moral activity, less to make rational or logical sense of the judgments people make and more to understand the field in which they are operating.[13]

In this way, habituated actions become the key to understanding care: the patterns that count as providing for others at the heart of moral activity. Following Varela, I am not so much looking to people's verbal assessments to guide my investigation. Rather, embodied habits—such as bodily comportment, modes of affect management, or physical markers of social relations, like the differentiated *wai* (hand gestures examined below)—provide force to the notion that different perceptual patterns are at play in a faculty meeting in Bangkok than are at play for a similar occurrence in Boston.

Take, for instance, the bow that accompanies one's entrance and departure from a formal meeting space in Thailand. This bowing is a physical habit, a trained acknowledgment of social groups. As such, it can be understood as a physical marker of one's recognition of the social body of which one too is a part. In meetings staged in urban settings, everyone does this, regardless of social rank, though certainly different styles of the practice are evident (which perhaps may be evidence of class habitus). Even if performed pro forma, such bowing remains an opportunity to assess the space a person is entering or leaving, part of the process of attention to the social body.

The ubiquitous *wai* (ไหว้) is another case in point. The *wai* is a polite greeting in Thailand, akin to a handshake, in which a person's hands are brought together at the palms and raised to his or her chest, chin, or even forehead: the height to which people raise their hands depends on the appropriate level of respect warranted by the relative status of the interlocutor. Unlike with the relatively egalitarian handshake, if a large differential in social status exists between two people meeting, the person of higher rank will not return the gesture.[14]

These behaviors are trained from a very young age. One often finds parents helping their toddlers bring their hands together to greet elders. Schools enforce strict norms of bodily comportment. This was illustrated one recent afternoon at my daughter's school in Chiang Mai. The first graders were sitting in a circle having a snack. The school day is long, and some of the kids were wriggling like worms. One boy made a move for the courtyard. The teacher quickly intervened, physically and verbally drawing his attention to my presence, an adult, sitting in the circle. "How are you going to go?" the teacher asked. And, at that prompting, the boy dropped to his knees and crawled away, ensuring his head never rose higher than mine.

These simple examples flag a trained monitoring of social relations that force, and enforce, particular aspects of the social environment to come to the fore. Those aspects reflect what is most valued, morally privileged, or socially endorsed. Relative status is essential, in terms of hierarchy and prestige. Individual body parts are also salient. One's head is the highest part of the body and the feet are the lowest—literally and figuratively. It is for instance taboo to touch another's head frivolously, and I am told one feels a great affront if and when that occurs. Some suggest this is related to the *khwan* being housed in the head, though that rationale is not as suggestive to me as the felt intrusion and corresponding polite etiquette. One must recognize body placement in Thai contexts. Bodies must become prominent to allow one to follow norms appropriately, such as excusing oneself before reaching over another's head or refraining from pointing one's feet at another person or any sacred object. You must bend at the waist and crouch so as not to rise above the level of an important person's head. You must sit in a collected fashion, hands on your legs or in your lap rather than folded across your chest or reaching over the back of a chair. You must *wai* appropriately in greeting and gratitude. These actions of the body are woven seamlessly into social engagements and indicate that following polite dictates is of utmost value in formal public and semi-private interactions. Perception is primed to enable their spontaneous occurrence.

So let me return to the woman sitting demurely at the side table during the controversial discussion recounted above. She too bowed when she stood to leave, crouching to remain lower than the leaders' heads as she left the room with her belongings and lunch tray in tow. She was clearly habituated to registering body cues, relative status, breaks in protocol, and so forth. So how can we understand the discomfort that prompted her departure? The woman's bodily comportment and her physical positioning placed her in a nominal role in the group. She had no leadership position and did not directly participate in the proceedings as such—yet her participation can nevertheless be understood at the collective level, at the very least through her supporting role as observer. The parallel between individual and social bodies suggests that the conflict in the room was akin to a lack of equilibrium in the individual body, a dangerous condition that risks the loss of *khwan*. The lack of clear leadership in the room could be taken as an indication of an unhealthy state. The notion of the social body allows us to consider the sensation of group membership in a physical way, just as one feels a cold coming on or the familiar pangs of a headache.

The physical aspects of social conventions in these settings invite an appreciation of the interconnectedness that group participation breeds. The positions and movements of others condition one's own movements. A break in convention (as seen in a power struggle between leaders) leads to a break in standard performance that, at least for some, could certainly be met with discomfort, particularly if we take seriously that such disruptions are equated with a loss of *khwan* and a loss of healthy functioning. If, as the "peacemaker" suggested, the concept of face is to provide an explanatory framework for this young woman's discontent, I argue it must do so in the context of the overall social body.

Face and the Thai Social Body

"Face" has been used for decades to describe the internal and external motivations guiding individuals to follow socially sanctioned modes of behavior.[15] Erving Goffman used the term in a universal context as "an image of self delineated in terms of approved social attributes" (Goffman 2005 [1967], 5). In the Chinese context, the term has been divided into categories of social face (*mianzi*) and moral face (*lian*)—the former denoting prestige "gathered via personal effort or strategic maneuvering," the latter an indication of moral status based on "internal and external prohibitions for moral behavior" (Yang and Kleinman 2008). Larry Persons (2008b) has marked similarities between Chinese *mianzi* and *lian* and Thai face, particularly in regards to *bun khun* (บุญคุณ) or favor-based relations.[16] Implicitly, these authors reproduce a strategic understanding of face work, in which people maneuver within the polite bounds of social interaction and incorporate morally justified self-censure to ensure their optimum level of social capital. In the Thai context, I argue the assumption of individualistic strategy obscures root values and their deployment. As Leela Bilmes has argued, "The importance of the group for Thais means that their understanding of face is collectively based" (Bilmes 2001, 207). The social body offers a way to augment the use of face alone.[17]

Poor People Have No Face

Only one scholarly piece has been written in Thai on the concept of face: Sanit Samarkangaan's 1975 article, "Concerning the 'Face' of Thai People: Analysis According to the Linguistic Anthropology Approach" (สนิท สมัครการ 1975).[18] Sanit's work has formed the basis for subsequent studies of Thai personality.[19] However, the most unsettling of Sanit's claims are largely ignored in these subsequent uses: in particular, the close links he draws among money, power, virtue, and face.

The word *nā* (หน้า) or "face" has several meanings. Sanit focuses on particular expressions that literally have to do with the physical front of one's head but symbolically refer to personality, persona, and/or status. Following a meticulous categorization of phrases, Sanit claims positive face terms reflect the attributes society most esteems, including fame, pleasantness, merit, beauty, and importance. Negative face, in turn, characterizes those who fail to uphold cultural values, whether through displays of anger, lack of friendships, unreliability, appearing downcast, having much suffering, or even appearing older than one's years (สนิท สมัครการ [Sanit] 1975, 497–499).

Sanit argues that the ability to sponsor events or otherwise demonstrate prestige is a strong indicator of "positive" face; indeed, that which gives or displays face most often has to do with property and expenses.[20] Strikingly, such displays of wealth are positive markers of social standing as well as moral righteousness. The same is true of all face attributes. "Crossing" someone or proving oneself untrustworthy are, based on the negative "face-based" epithets, among the worst behaviors and signify moral failing as well as social ineptitude. "Saving face"— that is, avoiding the tarnishing of one's morally indicative social standing—is paramount. Moreover, face is to be promoted at many levels—from the individual to the national—as evidenced, suggests Sanit, by Thailand's willingness to host extravagant international meetings and its (then) growing reputation as a hospitable nation par excellence.[21] Thus Thai physicians from abroad and their sponsorship of the Bangkok palliative care conference show a means of proving and improving face. And the nurse's silence reflects the stakes, including personal as well as overarching group risk.

According to Sanit, if rich people with position are stingy, people will not respect them and will call them "negative" face names (generally behind their back). In a similar fashion, if poor people try to display wealth or act as if they have "face" when they do not, people will laugh at them and gossip. In fact, Sanit claims, "Poor people do not really have 'face,' and thus they typically do not really have occasion to 'save face' that much" (สนิท สมัครการ 1975, 504).[22] A tension thus arises: are *all* Thai people subject to Sanit's analysis, or only those in a position to partake in the "face" strata of behaviors? What about those people who are somehow incapable of such "face"? Are we to understand their social standing as a moral inadequacy? Certainly we would not say, as those who equate "face" with personality or self-image suggest, that they have no personality, no self-image, at all. And they certainly also take part in social life. But "face" seems reserved in some respects for key individuals or, alternately, for people representing or upholding the identity of a larger entity (be it a family, a group, or a nation).

To deal with this conundrum, Christopher Flanders proposes a distinction between "personal face" and "social face." Flanders conducted a series of interviews on the topic of face and repeatedly received answers akin to what Sanit described. As he reports, when asked who possesses face, "the most typical responses identified such individuals as the prime minister of Thailand, the king, sports and entertainment stars, teachers, business people, those in 'high society,' and the wealthy" (Flanders 2011, 121).[23] Only when pressing directly in such interviews could he find support for the universal aspect of face he promotes in his work.[24] Flanders concludes that while everyone has "personal face," only some have "social face." The precise manner in which Flanders' respondents admitted to "personal face" is telling. It was only when "face" was said to mean honor and dignity *in one's role* that some people admitted, as did on respondent, "All possess [face] because society has made it that way. The joining together of humans—there has got to be the giving of honor. [This] makes every person want to have a part of that society" (Flanders 2011, 123). Roles in society are essential, as is the "giving of honor." Differentiating between roles and deciphering the appropriate unit of analysis for the distribution of honor is thus paramount for understanding ethical behavior.

The Demands of Face on the Body

A main presumption of Sanit's work on face is that people have different stations in life. It is therefore *relationships* formed with people of higher status that are most useful in Thai society, more so than the rule of law (สนิท สมัครการ 1975, 500). In this framing, individuals are responsible for forging advantageous relationships, and their ability to do so reflects their moral standing, while the maintenance of set group relations is presumed.

This need not imply that active strategy is inherently bound up with face. As with moral action generally, routine continuously embodies these parameters. In her study of Thai politeness, Bilmes provides insight into the sociolinguistic foundations of face conventions. Bilmes found that, whether the result of polite protocol or strategic angling, face is always geared toward "maintaining harmony" among the group (Bilmes 2001, 188). Disregarding the roles of the hierarchy disrupts harmony; therefore, challenging the social system has a negative connotation, and such disruptions are figured out of equations of healthy functioning at the individual and social levels.

Thus the social body is continually reinscribed, not simply through individual strategies of self-placement, but also through ritualized polite behavior. There is both the sensing of shared space, and one's personal movement therein, *and* the pro forma acceptance of the overall shape of the group that comes implicitly in the maintenance of social etiquette. One could say that the supposition that harmony and equilibrium are essential to health leads people to maintain an appropriate (that is, more or less dictated or otherwise socially sanctioned) role in the social body at large for the sake of health and well-being. Following Seligman and colleagues (2008), as with care at the bedside, one can say that some of these dynamics are a function of ritual-like engagement. One need not attend to the meanings behind each and every action, whether when attending to the physical needs of another body or to the overall needs of the social body as a whole. One cares, one provides for others, by performing the appropriate actions themselves; one maintains the social body as a matter of course.

Such practices of care serve continually to reproduce societal values inherent in Thai face terms, even when people might explicitly state they do not support such ethical terms. These values—group unity above all, in addition to wealth, beauty, and differential status as moral markers—are those of a stratified society. Roles in the social body here are inherently unequal. Karma and merit are the invisible roots of stations in life. Displays of wealth and indications of merit empower people above others without similar means. This type of structure "makes sense," has an internal logic, but challenges standard ideals of egalitarianism. In turn, scholars tend to highlight that which does not contradict their own held value of distributive justice.[25] The scholarship that has taken up Sanit's ideas concerning Thai personality recognizes the importance of social cohesion for "face" but downplays the "stations in life" also required. Face indicates merit, prestige, power—and "group harmony" demands those coordinates stay relatively fixed.[26]

The Genius of Thai Society

In the 1920s and 1930s, Thai cultural brokers often used the word "genius" to explain the essence of their society to outsiders.[27] In speeches to the Siam Society, presentations by Thais to foreign pundits, and so forth, "the genius of Thai society" boiled down to the simple fact that everyone had their place in the social world: in a word, hierarchy.

Metaphorically then, social groups (and, at times, Thai society at large) are akin to a body, for which *phūyai* (ผู้ใหญ่, "big people") serve as the "face": the face in charge of making decisions and directing the actions of the body that it guides. In this parsing, only certain people can be the "face" (or, perhaps more accurately, the "head"[28]), and others are left to occupy other "parts" of this social "body." Face terminology reflects that which is most esteemed in society, what counts for prestige.[29] When putting its best face forward, certain traits—such as fame, pleasantness, merit, beauty, and importance—are understood to serve the body best. And, as explained above, people perceptually attend to these parameters and physically register the effects of disruption.

Social positioning has inner and outer coordinates. Positive face attributes map onto some forms of prestige and correlated moral virtue. Relationships with others, often including providing for others, figure prominently. Becoming a patron, hosting a public gathering, being a good person, winning the heart of your superior, promoting yourself, and promising benefits to others are all tactics for gaining face (Persons 2008a). Larry Persons also describes how to lose face, including failing, being criticized or challenged, being the focus of gossip or slander, not delivering on a promise, violating the law, and being overlooked. These are characteristics largely determined by relationships and surface indicators that others can assess. But being a "good person" is not ultimately based on surface characteristics alone: the surface is taken as a sign of an ultimate virtue. Nonetheless, outer assessments remain of paramount importance: only through the cumulative accounts of appearances can true merit be ascertained.

Emphasis on surface traits and appearances has often been noted in Thai contexts (e.g., Van Esterik 2000), as has the esteem gained through outer calm and composure. As explored in chapter 2, this outer calm and composure as a surface trait is both the means to and an indication of equanimity, rather than a mask of internal turmoil. In the ideal, the truly virtuous let transient emotions pass in accord with Buddhist understandings of the nature of the mind. Theravada Buddhist ontological presumptions are also implicit in the limited distribution of authority in the social body. As I discuss at length in chapter 4, only a few hold dharmic insight; in turn, it is only these few who are truly appropriate for positions of power in the society. It is taken as a matter of course that not everyone can gain such insight into "truth beyond truth" (Gray 1991; Streckfuss 2011). Some are granted it by birth, with the luck of a prosperous family, thus making wealth and influence in this lifetime a surface appearance that attests to one's karmic state.

Ideally, leaders, as the social body's *khwan*, are ultimately virtuous, though everyone recognizes this is not always the case. Surface characteristics serve as a proxy, and a community plagued by dishonest leaders may in fact be suffering the results of negative collective karma. Although imperfect as a measure, surface characterizations of wealth, beauty, and placidity, along with functional attributes of generosity and trustworthiness, feature prominently in the attribution of prestige. But the elevated ranks in hierarchy corresponding to birthrights and other passive manifestations of privilege have, for good reason, fallen out of favor in contemporary thought. In William Goode's estimation, this is because of the ethic of distributive justice, commonly upheld in the academy, which takes it that people should receive social benefits according to the contributions they make to society (Goode 1978, 340).[30] What I am suggesting instead is an ethic of karmic justice at play in an array of Thai contexts, in which prestige and hierarchy, as well as health and harmony, go hand in glove. Although this may not be the only operating principle (and in a globalized world the ethic of distributive justice certainly finds purchase everywhere), this ethic must be taken into consideration in social analysis.

These hierarchical connections are felt. Exploring the elemental manifestations of hierarchy, David Graeber (2007) argues that higher classes are increasingly set apart from the rest of society. Through physical deference (avoiding eye contact, lowering one's body in relation to another, and so forth), conversational taboos, and all the small ways certain people are made out to be separate from and superior to others, higher ranks are not only treated but *perceived* as different, marked as special and deferred to as such.[31] Perceiving is not necessarily believing or advocating. But awareness of differentiations along these lines is necessary for upholding social dictates appropriately, and that awareness is trained from birth. As reviewed above, differentiation between roles can be understood, at one level, from surface characteristics: wealth, beauty, esteem, and the like connote positions of prestige and, by extension, power. At another level, these traits ultimately are presumed to equate with moral coordinates, including merit and dharmic insight. Harmonious group functioning, paralleled to healthy physical functioning, does not require equality. Quite the contrary. One would not presume the gall bladder could do the work of the heart. Although there may be misfires by way of deceit or cheating, ultimately surface categorizations function as a means by which to differentiate appropriately.[32] As part of the social body, perceptions are primed to discern along these lines.

This ideology contains a mixture of religious and political elements that in some respects are incommensurable. The "genius of Thai society" certainly reflects a cunning that from many perspectives unjustly oppresses more than it nurtures, and "harmony" and "social unity" are not only promoted but policed. Nevertheless, there is a spontaneous manifestation of the logic that I have tried to illustrate ethnographically. We may see a parallel in Thailand to what Graeber has found in the European context, then: namely, that "principles of behavior which once applied mainly to relations of formal deference gradually came to set the terms for all social relations, until they became so thoroughly internalized they ended up transforming people's most basic relations with the world around them" (Graeber 2007, 31). That is, the logic of hierarchy played out transforms the social categories of prestige into naturalized assessments of the world.[33] People perceive a world thus determined: their experience is part and parcel of a stratified group.

Care of Ailing Bodies, Harmony amid Discord

The relations I describe in this chapter are of a particular variety; certainly, simultaneously, other types of interactions and logics are at play in the social world. Nevertheless, the conceptual model I offer here is an attempt to make comprehensible to my readers processes that are often unexamined. The "social body" provides a framework for a particular set of social relations in urban Thai settings: the manner of assessing groups, the role of set mannerisms, and the actions and justifications that differentiate those who lead and those who follow. The concept allows a metaphorical representation of hierarchical social relationships as well as a phenomenological grasp of the embodiment of social and political structures in practices of engaging with others. In this way, I bring to light habituated means of perceiving as part of a collective, alongside the values that these perceptions, and their corresponding actions, reflect and continually regenerate.

By focusing on habituated patterns of social interaction and corresponding bodily movement, I have tried to bring attention to individual and interpersonal routines as an indication of moral life. Care—providing for others, whether individual ailing bodies or groups of people together as a collective—is part and parcel of living a good life. The analysis here tries not only to identify what matters to people, what is naturalized as right and wrong, and how people enact their priorities, but also to show that these coordinates of morality are a function of perception. People constantly assess social status, recognize body parts and the bodily comportment of others, measure their own actions in relation to others, and indicate unease in situations that break norms of interpersonal interaction. These perceptions are habituated and themselves largely predicated by social practice, forcing us to consider etiquette, hierarchy, and prestige—as well as understandings of life forces (*khwan*), karma, merit, and all else that ensures well-being—as vital to moral experience.

Theories of moral philosophy are at risk of assuming that the virtues, values, or rationality of the philosopher's (or anthropologist's) own society are universal.[34]

I have suggested that some scholars have failed to recognize certain values in Thai society and, consequently, have missed key elements in moral experience, because those values place hierarchy over egalitarianism, conformity over individuality, and at times condone surface beauty and wealth without shame. The "social body" as a term attempts to grasp and contextualize those preferences; moreover, by returning to perception and embodied practice, this phenomenological frame can give a sense of participating in such local moral worlds.

Phenomenology here should be understood as the training of awareness for certain kinds of perceptions. The early European phenomenologists, starting with Husserl, laid claim to the phenomenological "reduction": a bracketing of preconceived notions about the world, a method they claimed gained them a vantage point without external or historical influence. It was said to be a perspective on things "as they really are." But early social scientific utilizations of the phenomenological project found radically different assessments of "how things are" in other places, including time and being. So, ironically, even though the early phenomenologists' intervention into the sciences importantly laid out a host of presumptions that come to bear on "objective" investigation, they were nonetheless blind in a way to the influence of the process of their own investigation and the motives in which it was conceived—namely, a Western mode of theorizing and philosophizing that often seeks reductions (of the more standard variety) and solidifications. To retain the label of phenomenology, and have it mean more than the amorphous notion of "lived experience," we can focus on the training of awareness in different settings. This focus can also serve as a means by which to move such study into a productive comparative mode. From bedside routines to more generalized interpersonal and intergroup affairs, a phenomenological understanding of care opens up a route by which to trace how social and political structures get embodied in practices of engaging with others. And perhaps how the inverse can be true as well: how practices of engaging and providing for others not only constitute but also can change those structures.

As an explanatory device, I have linked social harmony to individual health. But discord certainly exists in Thai social bodies, despite the "care" shown in and to them. In Thailand today, long-standing factions are at odds regarding a host of issues, from the interpretation of Buddhist scriptures and their proper enactment in practice (an element of which is witnessed in chapter 2's contemplative practice workshops aimed at retraining psychosocial support) to the legitimacy of lèse majesté and anti-defamation laws. I want to make clear that the depiction of the "social body" here is not meant to take sides in such disputes; it is meant to open up space for discussion that sheds light on forms of resisting and playing with the status quo. There does perhaps come a point when analysis has to bracket the correlation between health and harmony. Harmony is clearly a value, harmony is clearly a practice; however, how this value breeds naturalized oppressive patterns warrants attention and action.

In chapter 4, I turn attention to the civic landscape. In particular, I look at volunteerism—as a form of care between individuals, as a national strategy of providing for older people, and as an illustration of the themes of the previous chapters in the social world. Thai officials see volunteerism as a key strategy emerging out of Thailand's preparations for an aging society, with the potential to serve as a model for other countries in the future.[35] Close examination of what volunteers do and how they see their charge opens up the trajectories of care at stake in these endeavors. Maria Heim says Buddhaghosa, the fifth-century Buddhist commentator and major figure in the Thai Theravada landscape, essentially offers a moral phenomenology—a trained way of looking at the world, perceiving the world—with therapeutic implications.[36] Yet there is a nefarious side to the social training of awareness. Why is there so much trained attention on hierarchy in Thai social worlds? This question can and should be asked everywhere. In Thailand, posing it brings a particular cultural history into view. Through variously organized efforts, we can see how the phenomenological components of Buddhist philosophy get morphed into power-wielding contentions in the social world, which in turn harden lines of delineation between people and turn basic forms of care into fundamental means of harm.

THE CIVIC LANDSCAPE OF CARE
Merit and the Spirit of Volunteering for Elders

One day I wore a new T-shirt over to Ying and Aom's house. It was pale blue with the logo "Bedside Volunteers" printed atop a cartoon picture of a smiling patient in a hospital-style bed surrounded by three figures, each doing something helpful: one arranging a picture on the wall, one sitting and talking, another standing by with a bouquet.

Aom took one close look at the scene depicted and just laughed. She cracked up. "Volunteers, ey?" she asked, incredulously. "Well, they got the patient right. That's right, a patient in the bed. But volunteers? They don't do any of that."

She has encountered many volunteers in the years her mother has been bed-ridden. Her impression of such people is not flattering. To Aom, they are often self-seeking people who come over and ask some questions about her mom's history and their care regime; they stay a short while, perhaps make some promises, and then never come back. Or they come back only to bring more people who do the same, time and time again.

I witnessed several iterations of this over the course of my relationship with the family. Volunteers and staff from the Older People's Organization (OPO), the NGO with which I based my research, would on occasion visit to deliver a present, such as a scarf for the New Year or a blanket for the cold season. Pictures would be snapped, polite words exchanged. Mau Fah, their neighbor and designated volunteer as part of OPO's homecare project, would always be present on such occasions. Mau Fah would also visit on her own at times, whether offering a passing wave on her bicycle or bringing along an unaffiliated group of well-wishers, like the time she invited a group of traveling monks to chant at Tatsanii's bedside. The family accepted her participation with OPO, but did not generally categorize her relationship with them as one of a volunteer—that is, they considered her more an old neighborhood acquaintance, and felt she was merely trying to funnel some resources their way through the organization. Though they never ridiculed her directly, they certainly did have cynical opinions about volunteer activities in general; whenever I told of some volunteer event or initiative, they would laugh knowingly and remark on how the volunteers seem to do more for themselves than for the people they allegedly served.

Here I argue that the actions of volunteers—as perceived, presumed, and promoted—reflect the ramifications of karmic framings of care in the contemporary civic landscape. (In the preceding chapters, I have laid out such framings in terms of rituals of care and interpersonal support between individuals, as well as karma and merit transfer at collective levels.) As with care at bedsides and in board meetings, habituated action in the civic arena can provide clues about the social training of awareness and the contours of the social world naturalized in lived experience. Volunteers form the backbone of the Thai government's social welfare plan for their aging society. But although volunteers have been vital to public health efforts in the country for decades, there is still a sense among many Thai people that volunteering is a foreign concept. Something about what volunteers do, and why they do it, is marked as "other." At the same time, progressive social actors—including those very same organizations working for change in end-of-life care in the country—are promoting a "new" orientation to volunteering in which personal motivations and pro-social action offer a civic engagement route to making merit. In this way, the "spirit of volunteerism" (*čhit `āsā*, จิตอาสา) is reclaimed as essentially Thai. In this chapter, to make sense of this complicated terrain, I take a close look at who does what in the name of volunteerism. In the civic landscape, volunteer programs help reveal the antecedents of that which is most important in care relationships at the interpersonal, group, and national levels. I argue that power struggles over what counts as beneficial action may obscure a common and enduring ethical map, based on merit and karma in a hierarchical worldview, that continues to guide volunteer work and civic action in many forms.

General Fault Lines

In Thai, the most common word for volunteer is `*āsāsamak* (อาสาสมัคร). According to the Thai *Royal Institute Dictionary*, the first part of this compound word, `*āsā*, as a verb means to offer oneself to do something; as a noun, it means a want, a need, or a desire. *Samak* is a verb meaning to apply or to volunteer.

Āsāsamak, as a compound, applies to someone who offers to work with the willingness to volunteer (*samak jai*, สมัครใจ). The term is generally deployed in full only in relation to organized settings, where volunteer involvement is articulated as such.

A prime example of Thai volunteers comes from the Ministry of Public Health's volunteer program, `*āsāsamak sāthāranasuk pračham mūbān* (อาสาสมัครสาธารณสุข ประจำหมู่บ้าน), referred to by the abbreviation Aw Saw Maw (อสม). Initiated in the 1970s following the World Health Organization's post-Alma-Ata global primary health care initiative, one could maintain that, as many people told me, "volunteer programs are a product of the West"—or at least of an international arena. But with more than eight hundred thousand Aw Saw Maw volunteers now in service, with a presence in every district and every village, if not every family, it did feel unnerving when people would claim, "Thais don't have a concept of volunteering."[1] Whether selected or "strongly encouraged" by a village headman, or assuming the task for any number of other reasons, these volunteers are tasked with the advertisement of, data collection for, and village interface with many public health initiatives. The success of the public health volunteers has spurred other government ministries to follow suit, with volunteers now found everywhere from the parks and recreation service to the police force. National programming for older people is no exception. Academic nursing centers, nongovernmental organizations, and a string of government ministries are all supporting the idea of volunteers as the first line of defense for Thailand's "aging society."

But in 2008–2009, Thailand's Aw Saw Maw public health volunteer program came under broad fire, as the government voted for the first time to pay these "volunteers" for their service. It was a nominal fee—600 baht (less than $20) per month—but it served to tarnish the volunteers' reputation in some circles and called into question the value of the enterprise in others. Of course, everyone conceded that many of these volunteers are poor themselves, and they give of their time and energy to fulfill the ever-increasing demands of the Ministry of Public Health (MoPH). From infectious disease eradication to family planning, volunteers carry out the bulk of the government's health education programs, as well as various surveys and basic health interventions. In the past, volunteers were given an attractive health-care benefit in exchange for their services. Universal health-care reform rendered this incentive obsolete. The fee was proposed to cover the expenses that volunteers incur as part of their service, rather than as a profitable salary. But some feared that the government's willingness to pay these people would only further increase the ministry's expectations and the volunteers' exploitation. Others feared the fee would become the primary motivation for many would-be volunteers, negatively affecting their job performance. Still others saw the move as more proof of the ulterior motives of government volunteers, citing the political aspirations and ladder climbing of volunteers in their areas. Just as this payment structure was announced, a volunteer program for older people was launching nationwide, and these debates were paralleled in eldercare circles. Following the example of the MoPH, the Ministry of Social Development and Human Security (MSDHS) also moved away from payment-in-kind to a monthly remittance—though at roughly half the rate of the public health volunteers.

An additional element of these debates was the circulation of a new word that came into fashion around 2004—the "spirit of volunteering." Proponents of this orientation to volunteering cast it as a natural extension of Thailand's modernization and development. According to the Thai Rural Net (TRN) 2007 study of the laws concerning volunteers and charitable giving in Thailand, volunteers were first present in Siam during the reign of King Rama V, around the turn of the twentieth century.[2] The TRN contends that these first volunteers were convened largely in service of the development of the nation-state. A classic history follows: volunteer associations increased as democratic principles took hold; participation diminished during economic boom times, but increased again amid economic and political crises.[3] But, the TRN authors note, a massive shift to the pattern occurred in 2004. The devastating Indian Ocean tsunami of 2004 brought forth a groundswell of voluntary forces unprecedented in Thai history (coincidentally following the UN-declared International Year of Volunteers in 2001). As a result, or so it is claimed, we see in the last decade or so an increased attention to and demand for *čhit`āsā*—or the "spirit of volunteering"—as the key ingredient in volunteer work.[4]

The emphasis in the term *čhit`āsā*, as opposed to `*āsāsamak*, is on the heart's desire to help others. This represents a subtle move on the part of *čhit`āsā* promoters. In the 2001 Thai Charter for Volunteers (*padinyā `āsāsamak thai*, ปฏิญญา อาสาสมัครไทย), volunteers are defined as individuals who freely come together to help society; sacrifice (*sīa sala*, เสียสละ) in order to help others; protect, serve, and develop society; and want nothing in return. These are threads that weave their way into nearly all Thai volunteer policies.[5] So all volunteers, all `*āsāsamak*, might then be assumed to have this so-called volunteer spirit, given their free offer of help in the development of society. But with *čhit`āsā* comes a slight change in emphasis, an attempt to distinguish among forms of volunteering, with the implicit message that the spirit of volunteering accompanies (only) the best type, the truest and most trustworthy of volunteers.

Much has been written about volunteers in the American context, which offers a productive point of comparison. Alexis de Tocqueville suggested that voluntary associations formed the basis of American democracy. Some consider volunteer organizations the hallmark of all democratic societies.[6] American popular culture depicts volunteers as people who give freely of themselves, moved by implicit Christian ideals or what Weber might link to a Protestant "calling" to do something good in this world. In their 1978 history of American volunteerism, Ellis and Noyes provide the following definition: "To volunteer *is to choose to act in recognition of a need, with an attitude of social responsibility and without concern for monetary profit, going beyond what is necessary to one's physical well-being*" (10, emphasis original). And while a specter of self-interest may lurk behind such efforts—and indeed, appropriate remittance is a key issue in volunteerism globally—Ellis and Noyes conclude, "As long as the basic elements of choice, work toward a social goal, and lack of profit are present, the other personal reasons why someone volunteers are largely irrelevant" (1978, 9). Building one's resume, payments that defray the cost of services, and so forth are all permissible in such a rendering of volunteerism.

But what of the choice and the attitude with which one acts? In Thailand, a nurse in the deep South "volunteers" for her department's end-of-life care initiative after-hours by removing her nursing uniform and visiting patients to talk about palliative care options. A community member "volunteers" to be president of a new association after she is "chosen" by her peers, and in turn earns a host of privileges and a boost of status in her new role. A group of Bangkok insurance agents "volunteer" on a day trip to build houses in the impoverished northeast as part of their company's policy of "corporate social responsibility." Obligation plays a role in such instances, with intention perhaps more in line with a socially induced idea of motivation (recalling Abhidammic notions of intersubjective influence and participation in the social body) than with an otherwise conceived notion of individual choice. And, in line with the appropriateness of following form, explored in relation to rituals of care in chapter 1 as well as in relation to legitimate intention for religious attainment in chapter 2, showing up and completing tasks without a heartfelt self-initiated motive to do so does not necessarily call such actions into question.

Understanding *when* motivations matter, and *which tasks* count, helps deconstruct differing Thai scenarios. Here Aom and Ying's volunteer can help make certain fault lines clear. As Mau Fah explained to me, families caring for an ailing householder generally must support themselves. Though she was a volunteer herself (for OPO, which, as explained below, is in fact contracted by the MSDHS to implement the Aw Paw Saw elder volunteer program in the urban setting), she expressed great disdain for Thai government volunteers, whom she saw as motivated by money, position, and power rather than altruism. In contrast, she repeatedly told me how much she admired the Christian missionaries and their forms of volunteerism, including long stretches of dedicated medical assistance and the donation of money to those in need. But, although she had heard of the new "spirit of volunteerism" movement, she did not feel the need to morph her own merit-based activities as an OPO volunteer into the heartfelt and practical engagements promoted in that idealistic movement. The activities Mau Fah undertook as a volunteer follow a karmic logic, in that actions are undertaken to increase merit on behalf of older people in need. But rather than physical rituals of care providing transformations of karma and merit, for Mau Fah and her peers, volunteer-sponsored Buddhist temple rituals, gifts, or fun outings were the means to such ends. I asked Mau Fah whether, if not providing direct physical support, such activities were a form of, say, emotional support. Answering indirectly, Mau Fah told me such actions constitute a form of social harmony. That is, people take part in these activities, enjoy themselves, and trust that benefits will arise as necessary. Wholesome alternatives to stress and worry are seen here as means of psychological support, as discussed in chapter 2. What's more, the larger social context had an influence on individual serenity, a relationship between individual health and the well-being of the group, as discussed in chapter 3. The implicit message was that volunteering to do a host of activities, even if not directly related to the physical needs of individuals, was in fact appropriate and beneficial. Which again brings us back to the need to take better stock of what is expected from volunteers for older people: what is done, by whom, and for what ends. Given the broad strokes presented above, investigation of subtler lines becomes possible.

Remittances, Relations, and Rituals

In 1999, the Thai Department of Social Welfare conducted research on the needs of older people and found that approximately 7.3 percent of people over the age of sixty-five had no one to care for them.[7] Compelled by such statistics and the growing threat of their soon-to-be "aging society" status, various government officials conspired to take action. They launched a pilot project in 2003, modeled on the public health Aw Saw Maw, to harness the power of volunteers to take on the nation's long-term care needs.[8] In 2005, the program expanded from eight provinces to fifteen; by 2008, it was operating in forty-eight provinces; and by 2011, the program covered seventy-five of seventy-six provinces, with a total of approximately five thousand volunteers caring for 30,340 older people in need. The Council of Ministers (*khana rattha montrī*, คณะรัฐมนตรี) approved the official expansion of the program—Volunteers Caring for Older People at Home, or Aw Paw Saw (อผส)—signing its existence into law under the administration of the MSDHM (or, "The ministry with the long name," as most people referred to it), as part of the nation's official "aging society" policy.

Aw Paw Saw volunteers are responsible for five elder people each, charged with visiting them at least twice per week and taking care of their needs as appropriate. Qualifying older people include those who cannot take care of themselves, have no caregiver, are abandoned (or "thrown away"), live alone, or are otherwise neglected. The program's official mission is to help older people without caregivers stay in their communities or families, to raise consciousness regarding the importance of caring for one's elders, to establish volunteers as "neighborhood social workers" able to care for the older people in their communities, and to "establish local networks or systems of cooperation between the government, the private sector, and the citizens for the care, help, and rehabilitation of the health, happiness, and spirit of society."[9] Volunteers must have time to perform their duties continuously, have appropriate maturity and qualifications, be able to read and write, complete foundational training, and have knowledge of caregiving before performing their duties.

The depth and breadth of government expectations for Aw Paw Saw represents a radical departure even from the considerable expectations of public health volunteers. From disseminating information and connecting older people to relevant services to providing direct home care, the list of obligations is substantial (again, to be conducted for five older people at least twice per week). Relevant activities include talking and advising; assisting with food and drugs, bathing, dressing, cleaning, and exercising; accompanying to doctor appointments, emergency hospital visits, leisure activities, village meetings, and other community activities; and transportation to religious gatherings.[10] In an in-depth study of comparable public health volunteers, researchers found that the Aw Saw Maw volunteers were incredibly adept at information dissemination but must less successful with tasks that required consistent and sustained interactions. This casts doubt on the assumption that volunteers are ready and able to accomplish all that is expected from the Aw Paw Saw program. Even in the United States, where volunteers have historically formed the backbone of important social welfare and service systems, people are rarely performing intimate tasks in other people's homes, particularly those that demand physical contact.[11]

Government Aw Paw Saw volunteers visited none of the families I worked with in the Chiang Mai municipal area because the nongovernmental organization OPO was responsible for implementing the program within the city limits (the differences in their protocols and the ramifications of such are discussed below). But through Bree, the head of the government's programs for older people in Chiang Mai Province, I learned more about the implementation of Aw Paw Saw in nearby districts. In particular, I came to appreciate how familial relations explained a great deal about how certain care tasks were accomplished in this scheme.

Bree is a chipper young woman from the northwest of Thailand, thirty-nine years old, with stylishly cut short hair, down-to-earth mannerisms, and a warm personality. One morning we gathered at the city's main public nursing home, where Bree's office is housed, in preparation for a daylong series of site visits. Our company included the van driver, a stocky man who wore rhinestone-studded sunglasses at seeming odds with his manly country style; Bree's affable officemate; an intern from OPO; and a videographer from Chiang Mai University, charged with taking footage for an Aw Paw Saw promotional video. The mood was jovial, and we headed off north, quickly leaving the city limits behind. We made stops at a local community bank and a master basketweaver's house, both components of the MSDHS Project to Prepare for an Aging Society, en route to a group ceremony and lunchtime gathering of one district's thirty-four Aw Paw Saw volunteers.[12]

As we chatted in the van, Bree's eyes squinted a bit as she spoke of her mother, whom she had left back home under her sister's care. How odd, she remarked, that she was caring for older people but not her own parents. Here she echoed what I had heard from many others in similar positions, from heads of adult day care centers to staff at nursing homes. These professional care organizers would lament, always with a strain, not having the time to care for their own mothers and fathers (and here they meant the physical rituals of care). Instead, they dedicated their hours to the care of others. This type of expression, whether voiced directly or hanging implicit in a conversation, was often met by an enthusiastic assertion from others that their work had a great deal of merit (mī bun yœ, มีบุญ เยอะ), reflecting the common sentiment that caring for older people, even if not your own parents, positively transforms karmic loads. Certainly, family dynamics and economic pressures are varied, and with Bree I never had the chance to explore the sentiments undergirding her publicly sanctioned admission. But then again, the assumption that I should or might explore such sentiments is fraught, given the theory of mind I am claiming most relevant. And, as quickly as the strain had come to her face, it was gone, and she again was chatting excitedly about her love of the work.

The Aw Paw Saw volunteers share many similarities with their public health counterparts, but Bree was quick to make certain distinctions. For one thing, the fledgling program for elders is certainly not as well known. (People would often correct me when I mentioned the program, assuming I misspoke of the public health volunteers with the similar-sounding acronym, Aw Saw Maw.) For another, most of the Aw Paw Saw volunteers are in fact relatives of the older people for whom they care. As Bree described it, these volunteers are often grandchildren or other relatives (lūk lān, ลูกหลาน) who, through these government efforts, are supported to do what they would want to do to support the older people in their families. She emphasized how this gave volunteers for older people "more freedom" than their public health counterparts to "follow their heart"—distinguishing them from those who are cynically thought of as poorly paid civil servants doing the government's public health bidding.[13] But perhaps more important, the fact that these volunteers are usually related to their charges underscores how rituals of care at bedsides—the rote, mundane work of providing physically for an ailing elder—are accomplished by volunteers who, by most accounts, are not imagined as taking care of the intimate needs reserved for family. They may be volunteers, but they are relations first.

In turn, Bree expressed her hope that the new Aw Paw Saw volunteers would eventually be well known for their čhit ̔āsā, "spirit of volunteering." I was somewhat surprised by her use of the phrase, as the term was made popular in the context of civil society efforts (and arguably more "high society" efforts at that). And she indeed acknowledged it was a new term, one that signaled a new orientation to volunteering in Thai society. In part, the notion that people are motivated by an inner desire to help others—a heart for volunteering—is useful rhetoric for the government to deploy to escape allegations that they are using volunteers as cheap labor. Yet it is important to understand that, in the government formulation, this spirit of volunteering is not in contradistinction to monthly remittances or the tǫp thɛɛn (ตอบแทน) compensations that come in the form of travel, accolades, food, or other types of remuneration for volunteer activities.

Program organizers regularly bring participants together for group activities—often a Buddhist ceremony of some sort, followed by a meal. On our outing day, all thirty-four volunteers in the district came together in the community's meeting hall, wearing matching shirts advertising the program, to make merit together: an event that involved speeches from community leaders, chanting, lighting incense in front of Buddha images, and pouring sacred waters. We then gathered in an outdoor common area to enjoy curry and rice, served from enormous vats prepared by the village headman's wife, among others. While it is possible to critique these events as a waste of resources, they can be understood to serve a purpose. Recall, for example, Mau Fah's summation of group harmony and group merit-making. Such events may very well be an overt governmental attempt to announce and thereby create social cohesion. Nonetheless, they may also manage to influence the "social body," of which everyone is a part and through which forms of governmentality are embodied.

But in the bureaucratic civic landscape, in terms of actual home care, another set of critiques of these programs and their promotion is possible. In my interviews with ministry officials, I was repeatedly assured that volunteers were simply being supported to do what they would ordinarily do. I was told that Thais are phɯ̌an bān (เพื่อนบ้าน)—friendly neighbors—who support one another through thick and thin.[14] And as we dutifully accompanied volunteers on staged visits to older people, as documented on film, that might certainly seem the case. We watched (and recorded) as one male volunteer washed and clothed an elderly man with a severe case of varicose veins, and as a group of eager volunteers were welcomed into the home of an elderly couple. What was not clear on tape, however, was that the male volunteer was the son of that elderly man. Further obfuscated, the group of eager volunteers was headed by the village headman, constituting a cast of characters that most certainly is not replicated on a weekly basis, and hardly suggests free will.

In the province, these are unimportant details. As Bree told me, it was readily acknowledged that volunteers are often related to their charges or are put up to their tasks through the urging of community leaders. Yet when programs are promoted in Bangkok, written into law, and at times underwritten by international agencies, the specificities of Thai volunteerism are lost. Taboos against physically caring for people other than your own kin become invisible under the banner of the caring neighbor. Personal motivation and external pressure are morphed into one, without concern for whether or why that might be appropriate. In this way, the promotion of volunteerism in the realm of eldercare may very well obscure root problems in the social welfare needs of the population. Although volunteer initiatives can harness a tremendous amount of energy and social capital, the actual caregiving realities of the population are often inadequately assessed, over-shadowed, or otherwise manipulated by the rhetoric of "traditional values" and other platitudes of Thai identity that form the formal justification and assessment of volunteer programs.

The Thai state fashions the nation as one family, with the king as father. Hence relations among neighbors are ideologically synonymous with kin relations. This is complicated by increasing urbanization. Face-to-face rural relations become strained in cities filled with strangers. So, in collective assessments at the state level, distinctions among different types of relationships between neighbors largely disappear, in service of an idealized rural social-scape that needs to be re-created in urban centers. And, as a neoliberal ethos persists, state-led social welfare agendas are laced with terms that push responsibilities for the provision of services into the hands of "volunteers," who more often than not come from preexisting intimate relations. If we play out the rhetoric of these programs, it seems the government ultimately hopes to support and promote a system in which even strangers can and will act as family. But for the time being, although volunteerism is a recognized form, the actions of non-intimates remains either at an information-dissemination level or in the realm of nonphysical care rituals (outings, temple services, gifts, and the like). Bree may be earning merit by organizing volunteers, but in the end, it is not a neighborhood volunteer that is caring for her mother in their home village, it is her sister (who may very well herself don the title of volunteer for older people). Simply scaling up a program "by the numbers"—one volunteer for every five people in need—does not in and of itself take care of each enumerated need.

NGO involvement tempers some of the issues in government volunteer efforts, but masks the continuation of others. As mentioned, OPO is implementing the governmental Aw Paw Saw volunteer program for older people in the Chiang Mai municipal area.[15] Although loosely following national strategy, OPO's pilot project differs from the government protocol in important ways. A chief improvement is their dismissal of the numerical standards for program expansion deployed by the government. Again, the government program requires each volunteer to take responsibility for five older people (and hence the number of volunteers recruited is a simple function of the number of people in need divided by five). OPO deems such accounting an impossibility that borders on farce. The majority of OPO volunteers, by contrast, take on one to two older people. OPO also claims a more "organic" recruitment and training of their volunteers, employing a volunteer coordinator who identifies neighborhoods in need of assistance and works to find appropriately positioned people to participate.

I did not do a systematic sampling, but I found no evidence of non-intimate relations providing physical care, despite the focus of trainings and the rhetorical aspirations of volunteer programs for older people. Perhaps there were exceptions. Perhaps the trainings will serve to change the nature of acquaintance visits over time and as need arises. But as Mau Fah suggested, families are generally expected to take care of physical needs. There are limits to the friendly neighbors to be sure, and these quickly become clear. Bathing, toileting, wound dressing: these are the purview of kin (or kin-like) relations or professionals. For volunteer work, this distinction is disguised by the great number of family members attending to older people as volunteers. And, in such cases, the resources and supports provided to family caregivers is certainly an important achievement of such programs. But at the policy level, as well as at the training level, these categories are elided: volunteers are lumped into one category.

In a similar vein, I found no evidence of training on specific ways to negotiate entrée into homes of nonfamily members. Such a factor takes on increasing import as wealth increases, changing the relationship between public and private space. The physical layout of homes affects how volunteers can and do help older people in need. In a traditional Thai house, the living area is in an open-air space. There are no walls to stop the airflow or the passing in and out of neighbors. In dense urban settings, this form of house is rare. Even without going to the extreme of the large gated communities, where large houses stand like so many impenetrable fortresses behind patrolled walls, one finds that with air conditioning and other modern ideals of glass and stucco, houses are increasingly enclosed. One cannot just casually talk with people as they pass by; visitors must physically cross a threshold that is without common precedent. Volunteer programs that give people a clear and readily identifiable reason to enter homes make everyone involved feel more comfortable. Of the countless trainings I attended, dominated as they were with physical care strategies and practices, no one ever mentioned the physical barriers of entering a home, though I certainly found that, on visits with volunteers, more informal and frequent visits were made to homes with fewer barriers to the street.[16]

Ying and Aom's family were not typical targets for volunteer interventions because they were not as desperately poor as most enrollees (and therefore no worse off than the majority of the volunteer ranks). They were not living pinched behind houses, with dirt floors, tarp roofs, sporadic plumbing. Indeed, it was not without disdain that one of the OPO staff members confided, on more than one occasion, that the family did not really qualify for OPO aid since they were not poor enough. Their three-story house told the story, and the hours of daily chores that kept the floors and windows clean underscored the point that those who needed help looked the part. The presence of family members who could and did contribute to the maintenance of their matriarch's body on the second floor was enough to overshadow any of the struggles that accompanied their lot.[17]

Nevertheless, OPO and other volunteers made motions to help the family. The public health volunteers (Aw Saw Maw) did their duty in the neighborhood, dropping off health education leaflets or spreading the word about new health programs. In addition, health researchers of various types had at times come by to assess their situation and determine whether they might qualify for additional assistance. At one point, I too tried to solicit someone to come to the house to change the mother's feeding tube to save the family the costly and time-consuming monthly trip to the hospital. Several trips were made back and forth, me the eager anthropologist trying to give something back to my friends, trying to figure out whether any of the crisscrossing programs for social welfare might help. I sat with a young medical doctor in charge of a visiting nurses program and patiently helped him fill in a kinship chart for the family, applying the anthropologically driven tools for socially responsive health care made popular by the widely selling handbook *Community Health*, written by prominent doctor and anthropologist Komatra Cheungsatiansup and colleagues. The following week, it was with great embarrassment that I learned of the program's visit to the family: how they too had sat down with the family, asked about their situation and took up nearly an hour of their time, only to conclude that they were ineligible for a visiting nurse to come change the old woman's tube and that a lay health volunteer would not be allowed to perform such a medical task. Aom was of course not surprised, laughing as I came to the realization she herself had come to long ago: they were on their own.

Just as the myth of the traditional neighbor finds its way into policy, turning family care into a broader social expectation, so too does the presumption of feminine caring guide volunteer programs. Themes common in care work scholarship around the world can be seen in Thai settings—particularly the presumption that women are "naturally" better care provides, and that care provided by family members is necessarily better than that given by outsiders. The roots of this dual familialization and feminization of care have social and religious particularities. Gender norms in Thailand afford women more opportunities for cultivating the skills of caregiving. Childrearing practices, for instance, are customarily performed by women and are often mimicked in care practices for dependent older people. Further, women are restricted from certain forms of merit-making, such as ordaining as a monk, and the work of care becomes a similar, though less effective, route to making merit, particularly for one's parent. These same gender norms may in turn create barriers for men to overcome (socially and psychologically) in order to embrace and fulfill physical care duties.[18] Yet necessity remains fuel for care practice, and particularly when economic resources are limited, men are as capable as women in providing physical care. And despite stereotypes regarding women's innate suitability for care work, I follow bell hooks (2002) in reiterating that women are not inherently nurturers; nurturing behavior is taught and modeled. But again, what in fact counts as nurturing is culturally and historically specific.

As volunteer roles are increasingly institutionalized, we might note what habits and forms are thereby reinscribed in the social world at large—and likewise note too where slight changes in habit and emphasis could lead to major shifts. For now, government volunteers and their aligned civil-sector counterparts more or less maintain key norms. Their ranks are dominated by women, with a ratio of approximately seven to three of women to men. Direct emotional sharing is absent from their visiting protocols. Group merit-making is standard. Rote physical care tasks are performed by close relations, and the demands of such care strain limited resources. And only the very poor are deemed appropriate targets for charity.

Presumptions persist in this landscape, both practical and ideological. From a policy perspective, the countryside is presumed to need very little sponsorship for home-based care. In this presumption we find the basis of an easy-to-deploy cultural ideology that does political work. Basically, the government presumes that, with volunteer-based programs, it is adding extra support to what is happening already. (These presumptions are propagated not only in reports but also in group meetings and conventions, wherein the convened social body often serves to concur and support the ideas of leadership.) So too with nongovernmental organizations such as OPO, which rely on the basic Thai characterization of friendly neighbors as the root of their work. And yes, many say that in the urban areas, this type of neighborly care is eroding, but the cultural presumption that Thais understand the needs of others and naturally want to help is maintained: a boost to this base is all that is needed in cities. But while people freely discuss the merit of caregiving, the more indirect and "magical" modes of merit are increasingly downplayed in formal accounting, particularly as instrumental needs intensify.

"Smart Merit": Recasting Merit for the Middle Class

Win Mektripop speaks incredibly fast, in Thai and in English. His English has a hint of a South Asian accent, reflecting the time he spent in India researching NGOs and various volunteer movements. When we met in Bangkok in 2009, he pulled up to the prearranged noodle shop on the back of a motorcycle taxi, wearing a neat dress shirt and black slacks. His hair was thick and just over his ears; his glasses were square and trendy. He was young but poised, a fitting combination for the director of the Khrư̆akhāi Čhit`āsā (เครือข่ายจิตอาสา), or the Volunteer Spirit Network, an ambitious group he helped establish.[19]

The genesis story of the Volunteer Spirit Network is one I heard told many times. In December 2004, when the Indian Ocean tsunami hit the coast of Thailand, many Thai people were moved to help those afflicted by the disaster. The outpouring of not just money and supplies but also of helping hands—people traveling to the southern coasts from around the country to lend support—is said to have been unprecedented. Corporations sent groups, temples organized caravans, and individuals went of their own accord. What's more, people are said to have experienced powerful personal transformations through these efforts. However, it soon became clear to many charitable organizations that this humanitarian impulse could and should be tapped in a more organized and sustainable fashion; after all, since Thai society "lacked the concept" of volunteering, there were few formalized outlets for such donations of time and effort (the hundreds of thousands of current volunteers notwithstanding). Although Win was in India at that time, upon his return to Thailand, the Khrư̆akhāi Čhit`āsā was born: an attempt to harness the "spirit" shown by the Thai people in the wake of the tsunami in the hopes of making a sea change in the culture of volunteering nationwide.[20]

The Volunteer Spirit Network is the umbrella group for member organizations.[21] Its three main foci are matching people with volunteer opportunities, promoting policies at the national level that support the work of volunteers, and improving knowledge about volunteerism in the population at large. Talking with Win, one gets a sense that although increasing management and coordination capacity is of utmost importance, it is knowledge, belief, and behavior change that lies at the heart of the network's work. The network hinges on the term *čhit`āsā* (จิตอาสา). Win acknowledges the word's short history and skyrocketing use.[22] According to him, the sentiment is particularly important for young urbanites who, because of the influence of capitalism, think only of themselves. Volunteering in this fashion is a means to pull people out of the "rat race," at least for a moment, in service of others.

Key actors in the network are prominent figures in Thai society. Chief among its supporters are the celebrated physician Dr. Prawase Wasi and the activist and intellectual monk Phra Paisal Wisalo, both of whom are quoted extensively in the network's pamphlets and other promotional materials. In describing early American volunteer efforts, Ellis and Noyes write that "progressive causes [tend] to attract strange bedfellows" (1978, 157). But the mix of bedfellows in the case of Thai volunteering in general, and the spirit of volunteering in particular, may force us to question just how "progressive" the cause is. At the very least, they certainly provide an important vantage point from which to understand the roots of political power operating in these efforts, as well as the key assumptions about Thai subjectivity dominant in elite circles.

Although Dr. Prawase is arguably more renowned, Phra Paisal is the spiritual leader of the network. Throughout the remainder of this chapter I return to Phra Paisal because his positionality helps identify persistent terrain in the civic landscape. He does not hold a position in the umbrella organization, but he is the head of a member group—the Phuthikā Network (Khrŭakhāi Phuthikā, เครือข่ายพุทธิกา), an explicitly Buddhist collective. One of this group's three major projects is the Confronting Death Peacefully initiative, discussed in chapter 2, to help combat the overuse of medical technologies in medical settings at the end of life and to encourage people to prepare for death with mindfulness. Those trainings include a volunteer component, with *čhit`āsā* encouraged by trips to critical patients in hospitals during the course of seminar weekends. Another Phuthikā project is called True Wisdom-Based Happiness, which attempts to help people focus on and develop the type of happiness that emerges from right (dharmic) engagement with the world. And another, Smart Merit and the Spirit of Volunteerism (*khrōngkān chalāt thambun duai čhit`āsā*, โครงการฉลาดทำบุญด้วยจิตอาสา), is a project aimed at inspiring people to help others in the world as a means of merit-making, spiritual fulfillment, and positive social change.

Based on training fees and enrollment demographics, these programs most attract the educated middle class. And with this population, the group makes a fascinating move to recast merit-making opportunities. Appealing to a long-standing cultural tradition, they essentially reinvent the aspects of the practice with which many educated people are uncomfortable, namely the performative, magical, or otherwise unscientific modes of karmic transformation. As described in chapter 1, merit-making is a pervasive and profound religious practice that defies typical worldly logic of cause and effect. For instance, a person makes a donation at a temple, but the act itself provides for a transformation of one's own merit, the merit of a loved one (alive or deceased), or the collective merit of the group. And whether in this life or the next, merit has acknowledged influence on social and spiritual standing. Not surprisingly though, not everyone is comfortable with the somewhat ineffable logic of cause and effect intrinsic to such practice. While such nonscientific elements of Buddhism have long been downplayed (see Tambiah's *World Conqueror, World Renouncer* for examples from the nineteenth century), Thai Buddhist intellectuals are again increasingly promoting the advanced scientific nature of Buddhism overall.[23]

With the recasting of aspects of practiced religion comes also a recasting of care and its constituent parts. I talked with countless people who were eager to explain to me that certain ritual practices I witnessed at temples were not "real Buddhism." Such people were young and old, but almost always educated beyond secondary school and of relatively substantial means. Many of these people were uncomfortable with the associations of merit and karma, though admittedly they did go through many ritual observances, even if only as "tradition" (and possibly protection, should certain "superstitions" be true). Thus, what the "smart merit" project has to offer such people is potentially very attractive: an active forum for merit-making, sanctioned by senior monks and justified with Buddhist scripture, which promotes helping others in one's community as a merit-making opportunity as potent as any temple-based activity. And although this does not change the logic of rituals of care performed at the bedside (nor the overall contours of the social body), the "spirit" angle here arguably adds pressure for a more "sincere" engagement with such tasks for them to "count" toward soteriological aims.

Just as Win narrated the Volunteer Spirit Network's story, Phuthikā members also refer to the tsunami as a key instigator for their work. The time is said to be right to improve the systems that support people to help others, leading to positive personal and social transformations. The narrative is compelling, but there is an element of statecraft embedded therein. The structure and history of nongovernmental organizations plays a part in its crafting and its power.

Governance, Stigma, Patronage, and Power

The Volunteer Spirit Network has three major sponsors. One is the Thai Health Promotion Foundation (or Saw Saw Saw, สสส), the major health-funding arm of the Thai government, which is financed by a major tobacco and alcohol tax settlement. (Saw Saw Saw's involvement is not surprising, as it plays a major role in all the organizations I discuss in this chapter.) Another is the TRRM, the Thailand Rural Reconstruction Movement. Although one of the earliest and most revered NGOs in Thailand (founded by Puey Ungphakorn), the TRRM has been criticized by more radical elements of society for its increasingly conservative agenda. Many see its current status, "under royal patronage," as most telling of its activities. Finally, the Thai "Moral Center" (Sūn Khuntham, ศูนย์คุณธรรม) —also known as the Office for the Service and Development of Knowledge Organizations (*samnakngān bǫrihān læ phatnā`ong khwāmrū (`ongkānmahāchon)*, สำนักงานบริหารและพัฒนาองค์ความรู้ (องค์การมหาชน))—is a public agency established by royal decree in 2004 with the mission to promote morality and development in the Thai population. On its board are such prominent people as the award-winning CEO of the Siam Commercial Bank, along with other leading public figures. The patronage of the Volunteer Spirit Network can thus be understood as primarily royalist, with a strong mandate for maintaining the status quo, despite its rhetoric for social change.

The social engineering involved does evoke biopolitics, as witnessed globally. One can read biopower in the Thai state's aging-population policy agenda: therein, aging bodies are increasingly defined by and put under the auspices of the state, which seeks to foist an internalization of self-help and community care onto the populace so that its rule is supported by the people "caring for themselves" in the name of good citizenry. Appeals for aid must be made in a way that casts one's body outside the typical purview of caring Thai neighbors. State recognition of someone as a helpful actor relies on a presentation of heartfelt motivation. But such a theoretical rubric, while very helpful for seeing rhetorical drives at the policy and programming level, is too blunt a tool for assessing the sectarian rifts and other particularities of the Thai situation. Ontological politics are at play here, and competing phenomenological protocols at stake.

The present structure and maneuvering of the Volunteer Spirit Network is a function of over fifty years of NGO operations in Thailand. NGOs are of course a potentially powerful force in any society, a force that governments have a keen interest in monitoring and controlling. That the network is officially recognized and sanctioned as such is, in part, a function of the National Cultural Act of 1942, which ordered organizations to register with the government "to ensure state control over a growing and potentially threatening sector" (Yamamoto 1995,

245–246). Again, in 1985, the government of Prime Minister Prem (1980–1988) initiated the NGO coordinating Committee on Rural Development, or NGO-CORD, "to bring NGO efforts into range of the government's radar" (Simpkins 2003, 258).[24]

In broad strokes, the establishment of the Culture Ministry under the first Phibunsongkhram administration (1938–1944) marks an important step in linking state structures with the creation and maintenance of national identity. Twelve decrees, or "Cultural Mandates," issued by that military dictatorship set forth a particular ethical code, linked with national security, complete with invented traditions and newly coined words that would become part and parcel of ordinary people's vocabularies and self-appraisals.[25] Further, Wichit Wichitwathakan, first head of the Culture Ministry and later head of the first National Security Council (under Sarit), promoted "traditional" Thai ways as a first line of defense against Communists and other "threats" to the Thai populace.[26]

As David Streckfuss recounts, "As with other newly coined words of the day such as community (*chumchon*, ชุมชน), society (*sangkhom*, สังคม) or public (*sātharanachon*, สาธารณะชน), *wattanatham* (วัฒนธรรม) [or, the word "culture" itself] was created for a specific purpose: to provide the government with a new system of control, a new way of arranging and categorizing people and activities" (Streckfuss 2011, 233).[27] Indeed, the Thai national cultural characteristic of a "caring neighbor" in government rhetoric today can be understood as an outgrowth of these early efforts to solidify Thai cultural identity; similarly, the work of the Moral Center, a public agency and major funder of the Volunteer Spirit Network, falls in this line with the mandate to promote morality and development in the name of Thai cultural identity. This level of discourse then plays out and propagates in group dynamics, as people police themselves and one another to maintain such forms.

Some groups choose to remain under the radar of such centralizing control efforts. In the 1970s, in the wake of major student uprisings and government repression, most organizations in fact did not register with the NGO-CORD (Yamamoto 1995, 246).[28] Why not? Political radicalism of various sorts, and its repercussions, is one answer. In the early 1970s, NGOs were a safe haven for radicals, but after the brutal 1976 crackdown on student protesters, which forced many activists into hiding in the jungle and sparked a major witch hunt for "Communist" elements at work in Thai society, most NGO activities were demonized and labeled Communist. For the remainder of the decade, "all forms of activism that could foster anti-establishment ideology were banned" (see Simpkins 2003, 256). Only after 1980, when the government offered amnesty to political dissidents in the jungle and invited increased participatory action for the "development" of the country, did the work of NGOs again begin to grow in the open.

The NGO-CORD has brought activists some legitimacy for conducting development work with the blessing (if also the scrutiny) of the government. But smaller grassroots organizations continue not to register, for several reasons. For one thing, organizations that register for official status with the Ministry of Interior must have an endowment of between 200,000–500,000 baht ($5,000–$12,000), and must create a board that is subject to investigation by the police. Although this process provides them eligibility for government grant funds, including the Saw Saw Saw funding stream so vital to health efforts, it also subjects them to fairly strict "social acceptability" standards.[29] So, in addition to the cost of acquiring the endowment funds (a massive expense for the majority of organizations), many NGOs forgo registering with the government to escape the conservative norms of social hierarchy involved. Board members in this formal process must be *phūyai* (ผู้ใหญ่), "big men," who serve as rubber stamps for the group's actions. Groups must choose wisely; these figures must be prominent enough to earn their group appropriate legitimacy, as well as supportive enough of the organization's mission not to halt important change work. This leads to what Simpkins deems "tensions between patron-enforced conservatism and patron-enabled activism" (2003, 267). Many groups find this a waste of time at best and an impediment to progressive action, and thus choose to find funds outside the government and work independently, often with funding from other countries.[30] But funding from foreign countries opens groups up to accusations of an "unseen hand" directing political work from outside Thailand. In addition, foreign funders often demand that groups frame their work according to international fads and funding priorities, leading to "mission creep": slight changes in focus that, over time, can lead to drastically altered engagements in local affairs.

Despite reasons for maintaining autonomy, the last twenty years has seen exponential expansion of registered NGOs working on an enormous range of issues, from AIDS care to water conservation.[31] These groups tend to fall into one of two categories: one that extends the more radical history of NGO work, the other with equally deep but far more conservative roots. The director of OPO once described to me these two categories as he saw them, using a pen and paper to illustrate his ideas as he spoke. On one side of the paper, he wrote "red," on the other, "white." The "red," which perhaps unintentionally evoked the Red-Yellow political schism heating up at the time, hearkened back to the specter of communism that had dominated ideas of nongovernmental work and political dissidence for decades. Political ideology may indeed contribute to such categorization, though the director made the distinction based more on the topic of work. That is, for the director, "red NGOs" are those working on environmental issues and women's rights. They tend to position themselves at odds with the government and operate with stridency and aggression. "White NGOs," in contrast, are those working for social welfare, eldercare, and other less contentious issues. This describes both OPO and the Volunteer Spirit Network. They pursue collaborations with both government and business groups and are willing to compromise and work within socially sanctioned modes of behavior to elicit the change they seek.

Social scientists have noted the red versus white conceptualization as well, albeit in other terms. Philip Hirsch (1991) described something like the whites as "collaborationists" and "culturalists," with reds as "autonomists."[32] The latter groups see any collaboration with the government as having too high an ideological price tag; in turn, they lack a vehicle by which to engage the state and often face resistance from ordinary citizens, as cultural mandates have been internalized and embodied as long-standing tradition. For the white NGOs, on the other hand, their status affords them policy platforms, wide membership bases, and political affiliations that serve to form partisanship around issues such as class, equal rights, and self-determination. The affiliation of Dr. Prawase Wasi, for instance, makes powerful inroads for the Volunteer Spirit Network in this regard. In the mix as well are GONGOs—government operated nongovernmental organizations. So between the GONGOs and the "hot issue," "troublemaker," "red" NGOs, you have what Simpkins terms the "social welfare/charity/service-oriented NGOs" (aka "white") that are less volatile and more collaborative (Simpkins 2003, 261).

There is a common misconception that "white" groups are a new phenomenon. But there have been links between government and the "third sector" throughout the twentieth century. The TRRM (mentioned above) was an early example of such collaboration. However, the political upheaval following the 1976 crackdown has largely erased such memory. In the aftermath of 1976, collaboration with the government or with the royalty often indicated a political conservatism that was suspect to many involved in social activism. Thus TRRM founder Dr. Puey's exile in 1976 and the group's subsequent reorganization "under royal patronage" have tended to obscure the collaborations it had previously maintained when it functioned as a more progressive development organization.[33] Nevertheless, some would call even these early collaborations deeply conservative. The casting of NGOs in general as a conservative rather than a radical element in Thai society is at the core of the discussion in this chapter. Although different factions appear to stand on different ideological grounds when it comes to civic action, even the more radical actors can be understood as taking a similar stage, performing via modes of action deeply entrained across social strata.

Throughout the 1980s, there was little state monetary support for NGOs of any stripe, despite increasing rhetoric for participatory development work and calls for collaboration across sectors. Simpkins assesses the situation as one in which "elites could have it both ways: NGOs could provide services for free (from the government's perspective), and NGOs' links to foreign funds maintained the servers in a vulnerable political position" (Simpkins 2003, 272). That is, with the memory of Communist suppression still strong, such groups were always at risk for negative branding and government censure. And through the various performative demands of the state outlined above, officially recognized groups had ample, somewhat forced, opportunity to resubstantiate norms of social hierarchy and deference in "social body" practices—such as organization legitimation protocols, board meetings, and so forth—en route to whatever their mandate might be.

Enter volunteers. NGOs at that time needed a route for attracting capable young people to their ranks. The Thai Volunteer Service (TVS, *mūnnithi ʿāsāsamak phǔa sangkhom*, มูลนิธิ อาสาสมัครเพื่อสังคม) is a historically important example of Thai volunteerism in the NGO world, as well as a key element in the development of the third sector in general. Again, regardless of claims of a lack of Thai volunteerism, the TVS has been in operation since 1980 and has served as an entry point for Thais hoping to work for NGOs. The TVS was established "with the objective of finding solutions to problems faced by development NGOs" (Pongsapich 1995, 255), including personnel, money, and coordination issues. "Volunteering" in TVS parlance involves two years of committed work with a member NGO, learning their work and possibly laying the groundwork for a future career in the social sector.[34]

As a result, volunteer initiatives today face the twofold issue of convincing people that volunteering does not necessitate the all-consuming two-year commitment required by the well-known TVS (in what essentially amounts to a Peace Corps–type experience), and perhaps more importantly, that volunteering is not inherently mixed up with the negative image of NGOs in Thailand in general. Indeed, a semblance of "third-hand" stigma remains for many NGOs, whether caused by an overly conservative or an overly radical assessment of their work.[35] More so than government-associated volunteer efforts, then, the Volunteer Spirit Network must contend with these historic associations.[36] What's more, these associations point us to real instrumental power footholds at play.

Thus, the presence of "big men" on the boards of NGOs is a necessitated practice. In addition to their effects in any given organization, their presence also continually resubstantiates the patronage system that dominates governmental and nongovernmental organizations in Thailand. Phra Paisal is one of the influential people capable of lending credence to the organizations with which he affiliates: in this case, those seeking to promote new forms of volunteerism. These forms are also of clear interest in the circles that have, since the 1930s, attempted to maintain social control through the promotion of particular ways of "being Thai" (witness again the Moral Center's funding of the Volunteer Spirit Network)—and perhaps continually resecuring the "genius of Thai society" (as described in chapter 3). To be fair, the Moral Center is not funding Phra Paisal's Phuthikā Network directly; and I do not have reason to suspect that Phra Paisal has ulterior state motives embedded in his engagement with the smart merit initiative and the various volunteer programs he actively supports. Nonetheless, by virtue of his role in society, no matter his stated intentions, he fits a position that remains open to elite-driven social engineering efforts. To understand further how this is the case, I turn to a controversy that unfolded on the pages of Thai news magazines and in the blogosphere after the violent crackdown on protesters in May 2010.

"Truth beyond Truth"

In September 2010, Kam Pagaa (คำ ผกา), a Thai feminist writer and public intellectual, wrote a provocative article in the weekly magazine *Matichon*.[37] In it, she criticized Phra Paisal. She went so far as to say his comments regarding the current political situation made her want to vomit. Her critique—alongside the passionate online responses to it—provide a useful springboard into the deepest issues at stake regarding the world of volunteering in Thailand, including not only the opposing factions and the institutional structures backing various volunteer ventures, but also the historical, political, and epistemological underpinnings of such work.

Kam Pagaa (the pen name of Lakana Panvichai, or P'Kaek) is known for her bluntness and for her daring. Certainly her direct attack on a well-known Buddhist monk follows suit.[38] She has "pushed the envelope," so to speak, in many venues: from her frank talk about sexuality and women's rights to posing naked and putting forward what she has called a "slut agenda."[39] Yet far from a mere exhibitionist, Kam Pagaa is a critical thinker and powerful social commentator. In this *Matichon* article, she used her dispute with Phra Paisal to touch on the most pressing political issues of the time.

As Kam Pagaa points out, Phra Paisal was featured prominently on the covers of newspapers and magazines with increasing frequency in the months following the government crackdown on Red Shirt political protesters in May 2010, in which nearly one hundred people were killed.[40] Phra Paisal repeatedly called for an end to violence and hatred, encouraging people on "both sides" (red and yellow) to "open their hearts and see the suffering of the other side."[41] Kam Pagaa's main point is that Phra Paisal's call for compassion ignores the structure of the Thai social and political systems that keeps poor people at a permanent disadvantage. This structural violence is a major obstruction to justice (including equitable distribution of resources, equal protection under the law, fair elections, and so forth). To illustrate her point, Kam Pagaa used the example of a poor rice farmer who has a disagreement with his village's headman. The headman realizes he will lose an ensuing lawsuit, so he has someone kill the farmer. He himself then presides over the judicial proceedings in the wake of the poor man's death. Kam Pagaa said Phra Paisal's advice is akin to asking the farmer's family to wait on the results of the headman's tribunal and, in the meantime "open their hearts" to the suffering of this village leader. In that political moment, the village headman would be Abhisit Vejjajiva's government, which ordered the military to take up arms against the civilian protesters on the streets of Bangkok in 2010 and then appointed the "independent tribunal" responsible for determining wrongdoing. The Red Shirt opposition group, the United Front for Democracy Against Dictatorship (UDD),[42] maintained their longstanding call for the dissolution of parliament and new elections. As the UDD had challenged the legitimacy of the Abhisit government from its inception, even prior to the killings, the continued stalling of new elections was, for them and for Kam Pagaa, further proof that justice could not be served with the government as it stood (and as it still stands, with a military dictatorship installed at the time of writing in 2018).

Prior to this *Matichon* piece, Phra Paisal had responded to a similar critique in his open letter to the writer Pakwadee. He acknowledged that, in the context of a recent interview, he had mentioned a quote about the need to distribute love freely.[43] But, he claimed, he also said that power must be distributed as well. He underscored how he frequently addresses "structure" in his sermons and writing, and thus he reiterated that people must recognize requisite factors beyond the level of the individual. Which factors? Namely, those that lie deep within the soul, such as attachment to self. Here Phra Paisal is gesturing to Buddhist philosophy and religious practice; from this vantage point, he surmises, people would necessarily see that violence solves problems only temporarily. Thus, with authority vested in him by his status as a senior Buddhist monk, he backs up his political point of view with the backing of *dhammic* understanding, with reference to the teachings of the Buddha and implied comprehension of the world at its most profound level.

In presenting this debate, I am not trying to weigh in on either side, but rather seek to outline some of the major points that arise in public discussion of this kind for what they reveal about the underlying dynamics of Thai political and social systems. Phra Paisal's biography, particularly his activist history, makes him a difficult figure to pin down, and I did not spend enough time with him to adequately provide testimony to his root orientations. But regardless of his aims, historical precedent implicates the type of organizations with which one might associate Phra Paisal's various initiatives, as Kam Pagaa indicates, and insofar as such associations are made, people may categorize their efforts accordingly.[44]

So, again, why rehearse this debate in the context of volunteerism? It is not necessarily to draw attention to the risk of prosecution that Kam Pagaa faces under Thailand's defamation laws, though it must be noted that there can be legal ramifications for directly challenging a respected public figure. Defamation laws limit critical appraisal not only of key individuals but also of the initiatives they initiate, including volunteer efforts. Recall from chapter 3, social harmony is not only promoted, it is policed. But also crucial is the use of religious rhetoric in this debate, demonstrated in Phra Paisal's self-defense, which, intentionally or not, serves to legitimize the class-based ideology and political positioning of volunteer spirit. Specifically, the impulse to cleanse performative merit-making from volunteer efforts has political ramifications. Promotion of a sincere orientation to community service in the name of embodied Thai Buddhist culture comes with the simultaneous disavowal of ritual orientations to Buddhist practice, found predominantly among the lower classes. What's more, common means of claiming legitimacy in such matters partakes in existing hierarchies.

Christine Gray has noted that Thai Theravada cosmology locates separate realms of beings, ranked according to "wisdom." That is, "Levels of the cosmos are identified with categories of persons marked by relative levels of detachment and hence wisdom and/or ignorance, and by distinct speech or communicative characteristics" (Gray 1991, 48). In Phra Paisal's remarks, he self-identifies as an advanced practitioner by alluding to insights attainable only via such "wisdom," namely, the recognition of long-term outcomes of violence and the obstacles to political harmony that arise through attachment to self. Historians of modern Thailand, including Nidhi Eoseewong, have pointed out that that type of wisdom is said essentially to be capable of grasping "truth-beyond-truth," a form of knowledge that is most highly valued and generally trumps other forms of knowledge.

In political arenas, this type of model of reality limits, by default, the number of people who can claim access to "truth" and, in turn, limits the number of people who can be suitable leaders of society. As Gray surmises, "Theravada societies are organized around a single fundamental assumption and epistemological model: that the *dhamma* is primarily a hidden or immanent phenomenon that must be carefully 'searched for' or 'illuminated' . . . [and] is open to a very few exceptional individuals in society—monks and kings . . . [and] men of pure minds (Streckfuss 2011, 67, quoting Gray 1986). This "invisible moral hierarchy" further maps onto classes in Thai society, reinforced by and reinforcing the power structure. People tend to accept that one's economic conditions are a function of merit; those with better socioeconomic standing are enjoying the ripened fruits of their karmic seeds, just as the poor suffer from their own karmic burdens. Social engineering has helped solidify such equations.

As mentioned, "traditional" Thai ways have been promoted, beginning in the early twentieth century, as both a governing and national defense strategy. In the 1980s, this trend continued as King Bhumibol was increasingly fashioned as the "Farmer King"; his efforts to make rain and otherwise support the people fell in line with popular descriptions of the typical Thai laboring in the countryside, a move that Streckfuss understands as a strategic enlargement of the king's royal field of merit, bringing an increasing number of people under his influence by way of this invisible linking of fates and a subtle manipulation of personal identifications needed to receive such blessings. Drawing on Gray and Tambiah, Streckfuss thus diagrams the hierarchical levels of society as correlated to ideals of merit. The "meritorious" include leading business people and the upper echelons of society; those "in the shade of charisma" and the "merit seekers" include appointed politicians, most intellectuals, some NGO affiliates, and the educated middle class; and the lowest groups (the "lowly meritorious" and the "demons") include most politicians, certain other NGO groups, and certain intellectuals.[45] These fields of merit, which assure certain entitlements in the social arena, are not bereft of magical or otherworldly components. But the modes of wealth transfer associated with the expanding fields of access and merit are not marked as such. At the surface group level, hierarchy is naturalized, as depicted in chapter 3. The Volunteer Spirit Network utilizes existing channels of legitimation and long-standing methods for inventing tradition, complete with the coining of a seemingly self-evident term. Thus forms of care get caught up in this politically engineered system of governance. Moving toward a more "sincere" frame of reference for merit-making, this kind of volunteerism may be seeking to revolutionize individual practice along an ideological axis that serves the status quo on the national stage.

In this chapter, I have brought attention to the ways in which merit is found at the heart of volunteer programming. This is part and parcel of what I mean by an overall karmic framing of care. Providing basic physical chores for others is care; so too is providing for the transformation and accumulation of immaterial power on their behalf. Both forms of care make merit, providing an enhancement to the caregiver's spiritual condition as well as a reflection of the karmic coordinates of everyone involved. But not everyone is comfortable with the more ineffable means of merit-making. What's more, dependent older people, among others, do indeed have this-worldly needs—hence efforts to incentivize people to make merit through tangible and direct physical care. Policy rhetoric generally claims volunteers regularly perform instrumental physical acts, when in reality they tend toward less-direct merit-making tasks as their mode of care. Such discourse may be understood as a type of "whitewashing" of certain merit-making logics, or an attempt to condition a sincere transfiguration of care practices in the volunteer realm that has not yet taken root.

To some, the economics related to unmet physical needs may seem a more salient framing of volunteer care. Some note that volunteers common in other parts of the world—those who work part time and thus have spare hours to dedicate to their communities—are difficult to find in the Thai context, where part-time work is rare. Some see volunteering as a mutually beneficial pro-social activity for those retired or without work; others fault volunteer programs for taking away what might otherwise be part-time work opportunities. Still others in Thailand explicitly envision increased volunteerism as a means for creating the conditions in which a large segment of social life can exist outside the economic system through sustainable, self-supporting communities. These varying opinions were expressed to me by a number of people, including volunteer project coordinators, NGO staff, academic nurses, active volunteers, ministry officials, and even ordinary people without much personal connection to volunteerism. It is impossible to categorize these opinions, whether by profession or income or other identity marker. It is nonetheless clear that categorical assumptions about the economic effects of volunteerism fall short of capturing the stakes of such programming in the Thai context.

But economic dominance, too, is related to merit here. Whether through classic ritual procedures or more "sincerely" oriented engagement in the civic realm, care as merit is a logic that interfaces with overarching structures of dominance that have continually reinscribed elites' place at the top of power hierarchies. The ironies abound, as those in need might indeed welcome the practical engagements of friendly neighbors, however heartfelt, while those in elevated positions solidify their status with declarations of such aid, however unfulfilled. Recall Aom's reaction to my "helpful volunteers" shirt: physical help would be great, but it seems, as of yet, to be unforthcoming. Whether orientations to merit or the provision of instrumental services will shift among volunteers remains to be seen. But this chapter demonstrates some of the means by which power structures find purchase in such potentialities. In chapter 5 I take a closer look at who and what the status quo of care in hierarchy serves to promote and who and what it serves to neglect.

THE VIOLENCE OF CARE

Pity and Compassion, Patronage and Repression

In this chapter, I work further through the unsettling contradictions of care in contemporary Thailand. My contention is that care works hand in glove with systematic oppression. The challenge is to frame analysis to bear witness to both simultaneously. Can we come to see how providing for others can help them in one way and yet injure or otherwise hinder them in another? Or perhaps the question should be flipped: Can we come to understand the ways in which people feel cared for by actions and circumstances we might otherwise recognize as harmful?

These questions are vitally important for discussions of structural violence. Paul Farmer built on the work of John Galtung and Latin American liberation theologians to popularize the term "structural violence" in social analysis and activism. Simply put, structural violence gives name to institutionalized, systematic, and injurious restraints on particular populations' agency. It has proven to be an incredibly powerful theoretical framework for making visible the connections between structural forces and individual suffering. The violence marked by the term manifests in every sense, from the symbolic to the brutally physical. The structural indicates the systematicity with which such conditions persist—between individuals, in groups, and through institutions—and the complicity of many hands in the erasure of suffering from scrutiny at every turn.

In formal response to Farmer's 2001 Sidney W. Mintz Lecture on the subject of structural violence in Haiti, Philippe Bourgois and Nancy Scheper-Hughes, among others, praise the importance of such work. But they call for further opening up of the "black box" of the concept, lest it lose its power and import. As they write, "We need to specify empirically and to theorize more broadly the way everyday life is shaped by the historical processes and contemporary politics of global political economy as well as by local discourse and culture" (see responses in Farmer 2004, 318). Where some suggest taking stock of different types of violence on a continuum to gain further explanatory and ethnographic traction, I suggest a focus on care: not only to achieve greater analytic clarity, but also to encourage solidarity and recognition of the ties that bind us all. Tracing the ways people provide for others can lead to understanding how victims become victimizers, how care can be violent, and how violence can be felt as care. As Lisa Stevenson (2014) poignantly illustrates for the painful and murderous effects of the Canadian state's "anonymous care," violence can be dealt as care; so too can it be received as such.

People's lived experience as caregivers links in various ways to religious ideologies, political platforms, and state propaganda. Religiously inflected elements of the Thai political structure, for example, legitimize and propagate particular sets of power relations, not only in state institutions, but also in boardrooms and community gathering places across the nation. These patterns exclude and oppress portions of the population. And yet, too readily calling out structural violence can disregard competing orientations to social forms, religious practice, and interpersonal engagement. Taking care seriously in all its manifestations allows for a more detailed appreciation of how structures are habitually embodied. This maintains Farmer's call to resist romanticism with historical, economic, and biological materiality: watching what bodies do is of key importance here. Care provides physical traces of larger social forces. The phenomenological approach I am taking is meant to make cultural history materially visible. In turn, it is my contention that understanding the social training of awareness toward different modes of providing for others may lead to novel ways of approaching social change and working for social justice, in Thailand and elsewhere.

Entertaining Structural Violence

In previous chapters, I have linked the value placed on harmony and equanimity in Thai social contexts to an Abhidhammic theory of mind and the karmic conditioning of experience. I have also begun to suggest that harmony as an operative social value serves to naturalize oppressive patterns within the contours of social bodies. The close correlation between care and merit serves also to reinscribe power hierarchies through paths of sanctioned merit-making in the civic landscape and elsewhere. Here I want to take a closer look at the embeddedness and propagation of karmic ways of knowing as a next step in understanding the pairing of care and violence.

Popular media outlets propagate karmic explanatory frameworks in a variety of ways. Although it is impossible to find a one-to-one correlation between people's ideas and the programs on network television or the content of dime-store books, the messaging put out for popular consumption does offer an important view into the social imaginary. At one level, we can find support for a phenomenological training of awareness, where attention to karmic cues provides the scaffolding for living a moral life. On another level, we can find the concretizing of social norms through karmic justification. When karma takes on this ontological quality—a proposition of how things are rather than a guide to how to look at the world—it can present a barrier to proper identification of both the proximate and root causes of social inequity. Parsing in this way, we can open a productive conversation about structural violence through an examination of the felt justification of the conditions in which particular groups are systematically denied access to resources, institutionally excluded from full participation, or otherwise unequally partaking in social goods. The tension here is between respecting alternate modes of social organization and recognizing systematic disenfranchisement. Again, the contention is we may have to assess both simultaneously.

Real Life Dramas

I cannot recall the first time I saw the nightly television series *Real Life Dramas 84000*,[1] but I certainly had many opportunities to watch it whenever I happened to visit any number of older people at 6 p.m. It is a captivating show. Airing on one of the main public television stations in the country, it is like a supernatural *America's Most Wanted*—with actor reenactments illustrating true stories of suffering as recounted by individuals, who are often in disguise or talking behind a scrim to protect their identities. The host, a tailor-suited man bearing a strong resemblance to Geraldo Rivera, introduces and closes each episode. With a thick moustache and histrionic presentation style, he dramatically underscores the moral of each story, with a reminder to tune in for the next installment.

The show resonated with many of the families I knew dealing with long-term illness. As I recounted in chapter 1, for most caregivers, the caregiving relationship was a case in which one's fate was being played out. At some point each night on the show (generally toward the end of the episode), a monk appears and provides an evaluation of the events in terms of *kam* (กรรม), or karma, somehow tracing the untraceable elements of cause and effect at work. Most often, the ill fate is a result of "fast karma," through which seeds of action bear fruit in a single lifetime. Thus negative repercussions of a particular misdeed performed earlier in life are often shown to be the cause of the suffering recounted on the program.[2]

Sriwan, the woman discussed in chapter 2 whose family shielded her from her terminal cancer diagnosis, watched the show nightly from her bed in her daughter's airy living room. Discussing the drama one morning, she surmised that the program could help you *tham jai* (ทำใจ), or ready your heart, for accepting what lies ahead. She claimed you could take the morals from the show and apply them to your own situation, and I got the impression she tried to do just that. She went on to mention "not getting angry," "not reacting to the behaviors of others," and "not nagging" as key lessons from the program. Incredibly, these all recall the "technologies of restraint" Maria Heim (2014) finds in Buddhaghosa's moral phenomenology from his fifth-century scriptural commentaries. Here in popular programming we find an iteration of ancient directives for healthy mind training, still cast in a Buddhist frame.

Although her eyes were often heavy with medication by the time the show aired in the evenings, one night as we watched she turned to me and, as if to prove the point of the show, pointed to her daughter-in-law, Jim. Jim had recently been in an accident that had crushed her leg and forced her to use a cane. Sriwan said it was the result of karma. Jim soon came over to confirm what the old woman was saying. When she was around nine years old, Jim had beaten dogs with a stick, and they both thought this careless and cruel action had resulted in the damage to her own body. I asked how she knew that past deed to be the cause, and Jim said she just knew in her heart that was the connection. This conversation immediately led to an even more intense issue, namely, the recent theft of a necklace from Sriwan's old house. The woman they suspected was a neighbor. They had not confronted her since the incident four months ago, and the woman still visited regularly. But their suspicions had been confirmed in their minds when, shortly after the robbery, the woman's husband was killed in an accident that cut off both his arms. "Fast karma" indeed.

Boonyuang, too, found solace and explanation in popular programming. As described at the book's start, Boonyuang, at age seventy, was the primary caregiver for her ninety-two-year-old mother, Grandma Maw. One evening, I pulled my motorbike into their driveway around 5:30 p.m. and found that Boonyuang had been lounging, perhaps sleeping, in front of her TV. Grandma Maw was, as usual, in her bed. I told Boonyuang I came over to watch *Circle of Life*, the nightly television program about destitute older people; but since that did not start until 7 p.m., I wondered if perhaps the karma show (*Real Life Dramas 84000*) was on instead. Boonyuang seemed relieved that I wanted to watch TV (rather than ask her a bunch of questions); perhaps she was also pleased that I just wanted to spend time rather than talk about or with the old woman.³ In any case, I followed her through the narrow path between a shelf crammed with various assortments of supplies and the old woman's hospital bed looming in the center of their space, around the fan pointed at Grandma's chest, to a chair pulled up beside Boonyuang's queen-sized bed, which itself took up the remainder of the room to the wall lined with revered pictures. (The bed was indeed an oddity in an old Thai home, but it had been her daughter's, and it seemed a comfort to Boonyuang in more ways than one.) She lifted herself up onto the bed and took up the remote, and we settled in to watch.

Boonyuang knew the evening TV schedule to a T, and flipped with ease between the three main networks, though I got the impression she favored channels 5 and 7. Channel 7 was airing a Mother's Day special of a talk show. It was nearing the end of the program, but it was clear the story was one of intense suffering met by model filial piety (*lūk katanyū*, ลูกกตัญญู), grateful children caring for their ailing parents. In summarizing the scene, Boonyuang echoed a sentiment I had heard over and over again: seeing people so much poorer and worse off than she was made her feel that things were not so bad for her. It was a compare-so-as-not-to-despair type approach, one I had heard earlier that very day from a nurse who spoke to me about how working with seriously ill and impoverished people made her feel better about her own life. (Such a sentiment may enable a kind of "pity" here that opens space to help others in need, as I discuss below.)

Finally, *Real Life Dramas 84000* was on, and it did not disappoint. The story that night started with a young couple happily making merit at a temple, when suddenly the man dropped to the ground. In the next scene, the young woman is shown crying outside a hospital, telling her husband's mother the news of his brain aneurism. And in the final of these setup scenes, both women are crying at his bedside—while in the corner, the viewing audience sees a green ghost of a boy about seven years old.

The next scenes alternate between testimonials and reenactments. The actual woman, speaking from behind a screen, describes her life as a widow; the next reenactment shows her leaving the funeral of her deceased husband. A childhood friend then accompanies her to consult a monk, who counsels her to perform a particular merit-making activity. As she leaves the temple where she has performed the rite, the woman sees her husband's face in the sky. He is smiling. So, it seemed to her, he was able to receive the merit she had made for him.

Unfortunately, this was only the beginning of her troubles. Four years after her husband's death, the widow is at a job interview when she awkwardly trips and falls just as the interviewer invites her to take a seat. The audience sees the same green ghost child run up from behind and push her over, causing the fall. Since the job was one that required physical poise, she is immediately discounted. In the next scene, she is crying with her friend and recounting how she felt as if someone had just pushed her right over. When she and her friend decide to go to a Tarot card reader, a wind rushes into the room and blows over particular cards (prompting me to ask Boonyuang again whether this really was a true story, which she assured me it was). There, again, the green apparition is in the corner. The fortune-teller can see him. She proceeds to ask the young woman some personal history questions, including whether or not she had ever had an abortion. (Cue dramatic music.) Indeed, unbeknownst to her friend, the answer is yes. So here we come to understand the reason for her karmic baggage: *bāp* (บาป, sin or wrongdoing) coming to fruition in this lifetime.

In the next scene: atonement. The women are dressed in white at a temple. The young widow is crying again and asking forgiveness from the child, who appears outside the temple window and eventually disappears. (The young widow could see the child, though the friend could not.) As usual, a monk is interviewed for the viewing audience. He explains the particular element of karma at play, and how *bāp* has been turned into karmic effects in this woman's lifetime. His voice rings out as the final scene shows the young woman in a meditation course with other people clad in white, all engaged in a similar process. And as the full explanation draws to a close, we are back with "Geraldo," the dramatic lighting and his soothing voice urging us to tune in again next time.

Just as in the Jataka tales, the famous narrative sections of the Pali Canon, wise ones decipher the meanings of actions. On the show, a monk is the narrator of such insight. In the Jataka stories, monks often argue over theories of right and wrong in each tale, only to be corrected by the Buddha, who casts light on past lives and thus brings the ethical ground into clear focus (see Heim 2014). Following Heim, we need not pinpoint an exact corresponding classical text for this show to fit and propagate the narrative teachings of the Pali Canon. That is, it is the *form* of seeking counsel from those trained to decipher past lives that deserves attention, the manner by which explanations make sense. Indeed, in contemporary practice, people often seek such counsel from a variety of persons—from monks to fortune-tellers, from spirit doctors to wizened neighbors—for insight into possible pasts. With such insight, proper penance can occur. Just as the woman in this particular episode can properly atone to the spirit of her past abortion, so too can others prepare proper ritual offerings or otherwise make merit in the appropriate veins. Of course, sometimes no specific explanation is sought; life circumstances arise, like a parent confined to a bed, and the proper actions of care become the route for transformation of karmic baggage.

Boonyuang denied knowing anyone who had ever been through an ordeal related to an abortion. But after our viewing, she again confirmed that she and her mother were using up their karma (*chai kam khǫng mǣ lǣ khǫng rao*, ใช้กรรมของแม่

และของเรา). It was, she was certain, her fate to provide care to the old woman, just as it was her mother's fate to suffer as she did. Only through such struggles could they rid themselves of their karmic debts, whether from this lifetime or past lifetimes. So the moral teachings of the program applied in general.

Grandma Maw did not appear interested in the TV program or our interspersed conversation. She seemed to be staring at the world outside the window, where an upstairs neighbor would occasionally appear to hang some clothes or pass by, leaving for an outing. She would sometimes use her working arm to lift her inert arm up and down, an exercise she had learned from a doctor and which she performed for everyone who visited. And so she lay there as we spoke, using up her karma.

Locating Agency

There is solace to be found in karmic frameworks. They seem most often to inspire positive acceptance of life circumstances rather than lament and despair. And, as Julia Cassaniti argues, karma-based models of well-being need not necessarily equate to simple acquiescence of powerlessness either: "The more one is able to let go of affective attachments, the more one becomes in control of his or her life and surroundings" (Cassaniti 2015, 180).[4] Of course, not everyone subscribes to the explanatory framework of karma, particularly as it is expounded in *Real Life Dramas 84000* or other outlets. Some young people I spoke with in fact bemoaned the loss of karma: they felt that older people held fast to a type of fatalism that allowed them a level of acceptance that the younger generation could not afford, as they struggled to make sense of tragedy or worked against the odds of the marketplace to get ahead. Nevertheless, notions of karma are far-reaching and subtly pervasive, even in the midst of ambivalence or disavowal. A sense of personal agency is less centered on individual will and more contingent on a host of factors in a web of cause and effect. But, importantly, karmic explanations in pop culture often trace current life circumstances to unknowable or unspecified antecedents of one's own doing rather than to systematic inequalities or forms of societal segregation.

Again, *Real Life Dramas 84000* offers a case in point. This particular episode piqued my interest because it dealt with a young person who goes back to her home village to care for her ailing mother. The protagonist of the episode tells her story with her face hidden from view and her voice changed to obscure her identity. She is a *kathœi* (กะเทย) or "ladyboy": born male but living a female existence, using the female polite participles and dressing in feminine clothing. The audience comes to learn about her struggles, and of course the karmic implications of her plight, through a tale heavy with moral undertones based on a particular set of social norms and the dire consequences of deviation. Early in the episode, it might seem a typical story of filial piety. Just as any dutiful daughter would do, the protagonist (I call her Madeleine) is shown lovingly preparing meals and tending to her mother's house. However, Madeleine has been struggling to find a job, and soon the mood in which she performs her duties sours. In the middle of lunch one day, she receives a phone call: another job rejection. Once again, she has been rejected because they do not hire ladyboys at the establishment. In anger and frustration, she slams down the phone. And then she proceeds to mistreat her mother—yelling at her, turning over a plate of food, and eventually abandoning her to return to her own home in the city. Thus begins a series of misfortunes that plague her for the remainder of the program. In the end, we are taught that her mistreatment of her mother was the source of her woes: the relationship with her mother, carrying perhaps links to connections in previous lives, was the burden she had to bear and for which she must make merit to atone.

No mention was made of the consequences of caregiving on job prospects, and little attention was paid to the physical and emotional demands of providing for another. What's more, no judgment was passed on the difficulty Madeleine faced based on the prejudice of others. If anything, her identity as a ladyboy was subtly cast as yet another repercussion of past deeds. Or perhaps not so subtly cast: a very masculine (particularly by Thai standards), stocky actor played the lead role, with an awkwardly placed wig and ill-fitting skirt. This can be read as a mockery of her gender identity. Though Thailand is often cast as an international queer safe haven, with traditional norms that allow for gender fluidity, many have suggested Thailand is more tolerant than accepting, and perhaps increasingly less so as popular discourse turns toward indicating non-hetero sexuality as moral decay.[5] Across the political spectrum, what might otherwise be a phenomenological orientation to the suffering of particular others solidifies into a karmic justification for socially sanctioned categories. These categories, in turn, can serve to limit people's social roles, as they lump people into stereotypes, script reactions to behavior, and even subject people to the violent scorn of those who hold themselves above such "types."

As popular programming repeatedly asserts that individuals are to find the causes of their unhappiness in their own actions, whether in this life or a former, it directs focus away from external circumstances that systematically cause or increase the suffering of particular groups. Although root causes are often untraceable, unknowable to all but a few exceptional spiritual consultants, they are understood as evident in one's station in life. What's more, the elongated timeline between misdeed and ill consequences means that a person need not directly transgress to suffer ill fate. It is completely plausible that a perfectly upstanding individual could be poor and unfortunate, based on past lives. But the poor and disenfranchised can take solace in this messaging nonetheless, as "true status" is not measured by education or household income: the good done today will be rewarded in the future. If those who enjoy power and prestige transgress, they will later be internally and externally plagued by sufferings due to their own karma.

The negative repercussions of abortion, certain sexual identities, and other would-be "antisocial" behaviors are a major theme on television, as well as in the bookracks at the local Seven-Eleven shop. Seven-Elevens seem to be on every corner these days, and traffic is heavy. Pailin Booknet is a major publishing house for this venue, and their slim paperback editions are updated regularly, with a seemingly endless supply of titles to grab attention.[6] Topics include herbal remedies, religious tattoos, Buddhist iconography, various supernatural issues, and, of course, karma. From the vantage of these dime-store volumes, specific actions lead to more or less specific outcomes.

When I found it on the shelf in 2008, *Chaokam Chǫngwēn* (เจ้ากรรมของเวร) was in its second printing. The title roughly translates as "Karmic Retribution."[7] The cover art features two flower buds and a butterfly, with two faint imprints of the butterfly faded into the background, suggesting past and future lives just out of focus. In a brief preface, the editor stresses the importance of such a volume. He warns that there will likely be a number of disturbances in society if people fail to teach their children and close friends about karma. Their "bad karma" will accumulate, to the point that the accumulation of "good karma" will be of no benefit. The solution, of course, lies in the pages of the book: these are tales one can pass along about the bad things that result from bad actions, teaching instances to help people see the truth and refrain from the bad. The first chapter is a good indication of the specificity of content: "Karma of Those Who Have Had an Abortion" takes a firm line that aborting a fetus necessarily leads to negative consequences.[8]

My personal favorite among these books is titled simply *Karmic DNA*.[9] The cover is black and red, with the contours of a fingerprint ominously impressed on the center. Its author is also known for his investigative work into the supernatural, including a collection of stories from people who survived the 2004 tsunami only to experience brushes with the paranormal. In addition to its explicit admonitions for people to do "good" and avoid "bad" in order to have a serene and successful life, the book also underscores the unavoidable nature of one's fate. Why are some people living a life of comfort while other, good people, are left to trudge along as day laborers? The answer is simple: differences between people can be understood as an outcome of karma (ราช รามัญ 2008, 34).

At first pass, we can see the broadcast of karmic consequences as threats, normative sanctions that serve to impose a moral order and maintain social control. What's more, we can understand them to normalize class distinctions and justify disparity. From this vantage point, karma does heavy lifting for hegemony, effective both for internalizing and policing, a means by which to uphold and spread the effectiveness of the dominance of a few over the many. But from another vantage point, these terms do not quite fit. As described in chapter 3, people certainly understand that, for instance, class standing does not always map onto moral righteousness. Beauty, wealth, and prestige are imperfect indicators of merit. Still, the karmic logic is stitched to a broader framework of following traditional dictates to free oneself from the wheel of samsara, the cycle of suffering. Ritual patterns are to be followed to enact transformations that one cannot think oneself into.

Ideologically, then, social conformity can be understood not only as a roadmap for right and wrong, but also as a form of care. Social dictates "provide for" individuals, protecting their karmic load and ensuring the means for their accrual of merit, just as harmonious participation in society "provides for" the individual as part of the group. One can follow the dictates of the social order as guide and participate in a supporting role for the good of one's self and one's group. This is the social body in sociopolitical form. Of course, such prescriptive norms are often read as definitive, without recourse to individual particularities. And in this way, violence arises as discrimination occurs and links of oppression are obscured. Nevertheless, without acknowledgment of the felt solace, logical sequencing, and dynamic entrainment of karmic justification, we may very well commit another form of violence with analysis. That is, dogmatic analysis can delegitimize a felt reality and risk dismissal by those who hold such commitments.

Arguing for a logic of care in social strictures brings with it a danger of being read as an apologist for repressive regimes. To avoid such mislabeling, I follow those who have made similar attempts to shed new light on Southeast Asian realities. Jordt (2007), for instance, urges her readers not to mistakenly read her work as a "sympathetic approach to the political status quo," but rather to see it as "a culturally *empathic* approach to understanding processes of political legitimation" (Jordt 2007, 12, emphasis original). Like James Scott, who marked a similar potential misreading of *Seeing Like a State* (1998), Jordt brings attention to something akin to internal resistance, but on its own terms.[10] She subverts labels like democracy and authoritarianism, arguing that "familiar Western standards" hinder more than help in bringing to light the intricacies of legitimation and participation in Burmese society (2007, 12). In part, she does this by laying out a "native epistemology" (60) and the relational basis of its corresponding moral code, helping her readers understand both the experience of meditation in the

Vipassana tradition and the political stakes of the mass meditation movement. Jordt thereby echoes Heim in calling attention to the restraint emphasized in this tradition: "Though social relations are articulated in terms of this basic theory of restraint, these ideas are justified in terms of a causal logic and not in terms of a normative code of ethical conduct that should be undertaken because a god or Buddha has commanded it" (86). The mode by which people conceive of and train themselves to be good people is intertwined in the social fabric through karmic logics of engagement rather than set ethical codes.

This is not to say that there is a uniform acceptance of an unvarying causal logic. And clearly karmic logics also can and do solidify into normative edicts. There are longstanding debates in Thai society regarding the appropriate interpretation of karmic processes, as well as the actions necessary to influence them.[11] And these debates too should serve as a caution against cavalier denunciation of structural violence along familiar standards, for to do so risks obscuring key variables in local equations. Identifying structural violence is often seen as a social science contribution to activist engagement, part of a quest for a more just society. I think that, for this type of contribution to be truly powerful, analysis needs to trace the workings of power without preconceived fault lines; only then can one identify allies and inroads for change. Indeed, what reads as "progressive" from a Western perspective may readily align with conservative forces, just as radical innovation may spring from "traditionalists."

Take, for instance, the progressive, or what I like to call "cosmopolitan," argument regarding Buddhist teachings, including notions of merit, reincarnation, heaven, and hell.[12] As a prime example, followers of the internationally acclaimed monk philosopher Buddhadasa Bhikkhu take Buddhist teachings more metaphorically than literally. Thus they understand "dependent origination" not as the laws governing lifetime to lifetime, but rather the moment-to-moment arising of phenomenon (see Buddhadasa Bhikkhu 1992). In this way, one might see "hell" as a caution regarding negative mind states rather than a physical place reserved for punishments in the afterlife. For those skeptical of reincarnation, this more psychological orientation allows their Buddhist practice to flourish along with other modern ideals of rationality and materialism. And indeed, Buddhadhasa's philosophy is a key inspiration for the international "Engaged Buddhist" movement, as well as a direct predecessor of Phra Paisal's Smart Merit campaign discussed in chapter 4. But in the introduction to Čhaokam Čhǫngwēn (Karmic Retribution, นพ นันทวัน 2548), as but one counterexample, the author emphatically dismisses such a perspective: "Heaven and hell do not live in the heart alone. . . . They are real."

Again, these debates are not new. Nor are they relegated only to the pages of karma books and the sermons of intellectual monks. In his 1986 monograph,

Place and Emotion in Northern Thai Ritual Behavior, Gehan Wijeyewardene recounts public confrontations from the 1970s and 1980s that echo the controversy of whether certain metaphysical contentions are to be understood literally or metaphorically. Wijeyewardene chronicles three very public, verbal attacks made by a former police officer turned monk, Phra Anan, in the early 1980s. In a campaign against corruption, Phra Anan directly took on Buddhadasa, as well as Suchart Kosonkitiwont (the controversial founder of the millenarian Buddhist Valley of Heaven) and Bodhiraksa (head of the Santi Asoke movement). As Wijeyewardene puts it,

> [Phra Anan] defends the alliance of Church and State, its conservatism and the popular practices which protect it and give it stability. . . . Thai Buddhism cannot be seen as a technique for individual salvation for an elite. Nor can it be considered merely the trappings for techniques concerned with the acquisition of power. What emerges, on the contrary, is a sociological view of religion and ritual, of politics and social relations. Things are as they are because they are conducive to the orderly conduct of social and political relations. To change things, to preach heresy under the guise of promoting individual salvation is to threaten this orderly conduct. This is an elitist view, because it implies that the majority of the population, in the pursuit of their own religious ends, contribute to the maintenance of a system that they may not fully comprehend. This elitism is, however, very different from that of the ascetic monk, Bodhiraksa, and the intellectualist, Buddhadasa, who in their different ways would remake religion to suit the needs of a small middle-class minority. (Wijeyewardene 1986, 31)

Wijeyewardene claims that scholars like Niels Mulder and Stanley Tambiah, who praised Buddhadasa as an important figure and unmatched intellectual in the Thai Buddhist world, were "too eager to take sides in what is essentially a Thai Buddhist dispute" (22).

Noting the elitism of opposing stances, we can begin to see the complicity of all sides in systematic disenfranchisement. Hierarchical social relations—preached in state-sponsored propaganda for unity as well as meted out in individually embodied behaviors—continually re-entrench existing inequities. But individually oriented soteriological aims that refuse the validity of performative ritual serve similar ends when addressing only the subjective needs of a select few. The latter seeks in fact to delegitimize the sociological conditions and meaning-making of those who consider ritual merit-making and social role adherence to be deeply ethical acts. Again, Wijeyewardene provides keen insight:

Clearly some Thai see their religion as a philosophy of individual development and salvation. They may reject much of the paraphernalia of spirit propitiation as so much mumbo-jumbo, and may even agree with Buddhadasa that alms-giving is some kind of confidence trick perpetrated on the populace. But for the majority, at every level of the society, there can be little doubt that participation in the religious life is affirmation of membership of Thai polity and society, and that all activity, however secular it at first sight may appear, is never too far away from a religious interpretation. (Wijeyewardene 1986, 32)

Wijeyewardene goes on to suggest that ritual in Thailand is not merely perfunctory: emotional well-being comes from its practice. Thus the "sides" are not so much oppressive versus liberatory, and choosing sides can in fact simply reflect the privileging of certain explanatory frameworks over others.

This all serves to show that structural violence must be assessed with an appropriate understanding of the structures at play. An underlying contention of this book is that structures themselves are nothing but habituated action. The actions performed daily in care are one way of bringing this into focus. If I, as a "foreign scholar," take the structures operating in Thailand to be essentially the same in nature as those found elsewhere, and apply familiar Western standards to mark the way they do violence to the weak and hinder the agency of particular targets, I leave myself completely open to the common accusation that foreigners simply do not understand "Thai-ness." And in a way, this would be right. For while, at the structural level, a system or institution may look familiar, at another scale of analysis it may be composed via different logics and different habituated actions; and if so, assessment of its dynamics and methods of producing change therein must be different as well. If certain needs are met and care is felt through habituated actions, however alienating or oppressive, alternative modes of meeting those needs must be considered as part of designs to disrupt the status quo. Indeed, if agency is contingent on one's own actions as well as the actions of others, eliminating structural violence becomes more clearly a group responsibility—or, more precisely, a group practice.

Pity

The relationship between care and structural violence unfolds with an ecological appreciation of the long-standing tensions and the karmic motivations playing out under the surface of prosocial actions like volunteering. The spirit of volunteerism movement—amid similarly egalitarian social volunteer programming efforts like those of OPO—seem poised to eradicate the more performative or magical modes of merit accrual in favor of this-worldly instrumental supports; but not only does this index enduring elite power struggles: pulling on this thread reveals webs of challenging associations operating in the ways people are providing for one another. The common sense behind many care acts is imbued with markers of differential status, which invites investigation of pity and its intimate links with compassionate action.

"Thai people are very helpful, but they don't like to be forced,"[13] said Brapin, one of OPO's first volunteers. Her candid comments regarding pity and volunteer work help make clear how working interpretations of Theravada philosophy play out along social lines. In her fourth year of volunteering for older people in her community, Brapin is also a volunteer in several other realms as well, dedicating one or two days per week at a local home for the disabled and serving as an active member of her district's Elder Person Club. Sixty-eight years old, this retired government worker and former track athlete now has time to use her ample energy in the community. And use it she certainly does. In her capacity as an OPO volunteer, Brapin makes regular visits to two octogenarians. As she characterizes them, one is a woman "with a bad leg," and the other is a mute, diabetic man with poor hearing. She visits them about twice a month, more often if they are ill. Visits generally involve casual talking, peppered with recommendations of various sorts. Because the old man has diabetes, for instance, she advises him to stop eating sticky rice.

Brapin describes her volunteer visits as difficult. As I heard from others, visiting older people is not without its unique problems and, despite general reports about the "good feeling" one gets from the interactions, these visits can be frustrating and even disheartening. Older people cannot follow the story when you talk, they do not remember you have been to see them, they are in poor spirits, and they criticize you. Brapin repeatedly says she "pities" (songsān, สงสาร) them. Nevertheless, she definitely speaks positively about this work. She says it fills her heart and makes her feel she has kwāmmēttā (ความเมตตา)—a term generally translated as loving-kindness or compassion. Thus a tension permeates Brapin's account. What is the relationship between pity and compassion for her and her like-minded volunteers? Answering this query sheds light on the personal and social stakes of one's orientation to volunteer efforts and care more generally.

With her fellow volunteers, Brapin participates in monthly training sessions, attends meetings of various committees, joins in merit-making ceremonies and OPO visits to present gifts to clients, and takes part in group outings, both those organized as pleasure trips for older people in need and those designed as a thank-you to volunteers and staff. There are, in fact, so many opportunities and commitments for volunteers that one might wonder when they have time to visit with the older people they are said to serve. Reflecting on her peers in regard to overall service, Brapin surmises that only about 60 percent of volunteers work sincerely "with conviction."[14] (Of note, she did not use the term *čhit`āsā* [จิตอาสา], but rather *duayjai* and *dtangjai* [ด้วยใจ and ตั้งใจ], more common words for expressing conviction, sincerity, or attentiveness.) She feels that nearly half of volunteers participate only for the socializing and congratulations, and do not do their proper duty for the older people for whom they are responsible. Moreover, not everyone does all they say they do. There are reporting procedures, forms with which every volunteer reports the frequency of their visits and aid activities, but there are problems with the system. Reviewing one volunteer's records, it hardly seemed possible that she had visited seven people every day since the program's inception, and the director of OPO freely acknowledges some people exaggerate their work.

Many people offered me theories of volunteerism during my fieldwork. For instance, one male OPO volunteer, a retired government worker who was nearly eighty years old himself, told me there are three types of volunteers: those who work selflessly for others without wanting anything in return, those who work for praise, and those who participate not only for praise but for more tangible compensation as well. Brapin would most likely agree with such a parsing, as she told me she would like to see a recruiting system that accepts only those willing and able to provide services to others without needing anything themselves. And in part, this means those who are in a slightly elevated social class.

Brapin explicitly denied that poor people are incapable of being good volunteers. However, she did say that, to be truly effective, one needed not only to have time to lend, but also be of higher social standing than those being served. In part, this was about having the ability to do for others without "looking out for their next meal" at the same time. In this way, she intimated that many volunteers were interested in benefits and incentives, both out of a vanity of sorts and out of necessity. But there was more to her class-based assertion. In the context of a visit, Brapin believed that older people are most encouraged by a visit from someone of elevated status. (Status could be elevated economically or spiritually: often overlapping but nonetheless distinct categories.) She said if a person of equal or poorer stature comes to visit, the older person will "not believe" them. So she outright claims that people of lower position "believe," trust, and are helped by volunteers of relatively higher position. She attributes the fact that the diabetic man she visits does not alter his eating habits, at her suggestion, to his inability to *hear* her, maintaining that their relative statures create the necessary alchemy to produce positive behavior change in general.[15]

A class effect is clear in most volunteer relations. Most formal volunteers are still drawn from the lower echelons of society, despite the Volunteer Spirit Network's efforts to attract upper- and middle-class people to volunteering. But even among poor people, class divisions come to bear on charitable interactions, though to what end is not completely discernable from self-reports like Brapin's. First, I suspect that certain presumptions regarding the immediate respect garnered by higher status are inflated at best. But further, consider the physical comportment of deference necessitated by differential status in Thai cultural norms described in chapter 3—even the height of one's automatic *wai* gesture of greeting is contingent on and reflects status, physically situating people in relation to one another. The social body functions in a hierarchical mode, enabling care to flow legibly in some directions and not others. The main point here is to add another measure of caution to meta-level claims regarding people helping one another at the grassroots level. As much as humanitarian promoters of volunteer-based initiatives might like to assume parity, there is in fact often disparity built into these systems in one way or another.

This all relates back to the role of "pity." Brapin is certainly not alone in her use of "pity" as a motivation for charitable action. Many people talked with me about the importance of pity, a force they saw as necessary for compelling people to help others. Pity also plays a part in popular fund-raising efforts. Take, for instance, the well-known Thai television program *Circle of Life* (*wongwīan chīwit*, วงเวียนชีวิต). Each week, it features a destitute older person. Details of their lives are provided, with cameras searching through every nook and cranny of their poverty-stricken existence (literally panning over dirt floors and behind makeshift partitions), with abject subjects depicted without any prospect of bettering their circumstances. In contrast, I think it fair to say that in the United States it is generally understood that to elicit charity, people need to be depicted as trying to help themselves and thus worthy of help to get "back on their feet." In Thailand, no such standard seems to apply. The circumstances that have befallen an individual, generally no matter the proximate cause, elicit the necessary pity. Ultimate cause and effect are found in equations of karma and merit that span lifetimes. Money pours in from around the country in response to those on the program—abandoned, helpless, and penniless.

Brapin explicitly linked this type of pity with the Buddhist principle of *mēttā* (เมตตา)[16] As we discussed her volunteer work, Brapin used the word *mēttā* to explain how she felt when she saw older people in need, or when she visited the home for the disabled, and so forth.[17] Given common translations for the terms in Buddhist studies and international communities of practice, I assumed she meant something like "love" when she said *mēttā*. So I was shocked when, after I asked her what the term meant, she said "pity" (*songsān*). She explained that, in Buddhism, *mēttā* and *karunā* (กรุณา) are essential to charity: *mēttā*, for her, meaning pity and *karunā* meaning the desire for others to be happy. Translation of terms can always leave room for misconstrual, but the underlying question about the role of "pity" in compassion remains: Does expression of sorrow for the misfortunes of others also imply the inferiority (in some way or another) of those pitied?[18] And if so, even if just in practice, is systemic inferiority a component of society and its social values?

As implied throughout this book, a broad introductory understanding of basic Buddhist tenets across traditions might ordinarily yield (however fraught) the following synopsis: The Buddha preached impermanence.[19] Suffering is caused by attachment, itself a function of ignorance of the transient nature of things. And comprehension of this basic truth of impermanence leads to compassion: a pull to eliminate suffering, with clarity about its root causes (namely, worldly attachment).[20] So when Brapin refers to *mēttā*, she is invoking the four sublime states (generally translated as love, compassion, sympathetic joy, and equanimity) that reflect ideal conduct in the transient world. Of course, Brapin may just have a fundamental misunderstanding of these Buddhist teachings. (But to be clear, I am not trying to analyze authentic "Buddhist" compassion here.) The point is that the prevalence with which I heard this equation—pity as a virtue undergirding charitable action—indicates to me it illustrates an important correlation in popular consciousness. Getting at the specific origins of the pity-compassion equation in Thailand may be fundamental to appraisals of social hierarchy and care alike.

A philosophical diversion is necessary to make this clear. How does anyone recognize the suffering of others (and thus be moved to act in response)? Edith Stein took up this fundamental question in 1917 in *On the Problem of Empathy.*[21] Stein comes to define empathy as the capacity to recognize others at all. So where her teacher, Husserl, assumed that there were other "I"s (consciousnesses foreign to oneself), Stein asked, how does one know that? Thus, empathy, in her parsing, is not so much a sense constituted out of experience but an innate capacity.[22] This recalls the popular Thai idiom: `ao jai khao mā sai jai rao` (เอาใจเขามาใส่ใจเรา), "the wants and needs of others come into our heart." That no one during my field research could really ever articulate *how* you perform this intuitive act makes sense according to Stein—it is akin to knowing that we live amid other living beings, separate from us, who have their own perspectives and are perhaps only partially knowable, but knowable somehow, through this empathic capacity.[23]

But again, in Thailand, what follows, or what should follow such an empathic understanding, is duty-bound, according to cultural parameters. As I have suggested in previous chapters, in general one should seek to take a friend's mind off their trouble, one should "make merit" to combat tragedy or illness, one should maintain harmonious surface relations despite fundamental disagreements. Of course, culture is not static, and as has always been the case, the parameters of appropriate conduct are in constant negotiation. Indeed, the volunteer spirit movement is banking on this malleability of norms and orientations.

Analytically, we can situate empathy as a precursor to compassion: the capacity of understanding another (empathy) then tends toward compassion (a feeling for another that moves one to try to alleviate their suffering). So in regard to Brapin and the role of pity, what does it mean for benevolence to be linked to pity? And can the two, together, count as compassionate action in social analyses? Brapin suggested pity as a "mediating" element between what I am calling empathy, the recognition of another's suffering, and the move to act on another's behalf. My suspicion is that, when the elements are linked in this way, social scientific analyses tend to question the authenticity of action, revealing a bias toward egalitarianism as the only legitimate form of social cohesion. If, instead, we accept the correlation (with suspended judgment), a more nuanced analysis is possible. A hierarchical society provides a system by which to identify the pitiable, and thus those who are worthy of help. With pity bound up with differential status, care and the appropriate means of providing for others become inherently bound up with social patterning. As I described in chapter 4, concerted efforts to define such patterning have been ongoing throughout the twentieth century in Thailand. Pity is in some ways unproblematic when social hierarchy naturalizes rank and privation.[24]

According to the director of OPO, there is indeed a "social norm" among Thais to donate to those who are pitiable (*nā songsān*, น่าสงสาร); however, it is his intention for the work of his organization to fight against such a norm. He wants his volunteers to feel they are working *together* with older people—and in fact *not* to pity them (*mai tǭng songsān*, ไม่ต้องสงสาร). I asked if he thought it was working, to which he replied, "I don't know, but I keep telling them."

For the director of OPO, there are certainly international funding streams that discourage the association of development work with "pity," and that instead encourage him to see "empowerment" as the key to program success. Similarly, the more "organic" modes of organizing seen in the volunteer spirit movement promote similar ideals, at least on the individual level, if not over the social hierarchy as a whole. (One could even locate the Phuthikā Network's Confronting Death Peacefully role-plays on a similar axis.) But those who, like the director, seek to eradicate a pity connection and encourage participatory action are fighting powerful social norms. What's more, their work to motivate, train, and promote the work of volunteers in practice does little to eradicate the connection between pity and compassion. Indeed, as described in the structures of organization and promotion that the Volunteer Spirit Network utilizes, class hierarchy is arguably reinforced on multiple levels in such schemes. From Aom and Ying not appearing downtrodden enough for aid to the subtle downgrading of performative merit traditions, a radical reorientation to social equality is not yet detectable. In any case, Brapin at least has not yet gotten the message. For her, volunteering harnesses the mechanism by which people act for others: namely, a feeling of pity that arises for those less fortunate and guides action. In fact, if obligation is imposed, charity breaks down; after all, as she told me, "Thais don't like to be forced."

Habituation to the social world may take the feeling of being forced out of the equation, essentially masking the effects of power dynamics through the phenomenological training of awareness. As argued in chapter 3, perception is contingent on how we move through the world; what stands out as important in the social environment is a function of norms, which become naturalized through repetition. In noting the rhetorical uses of Buddhist philosophy in this regard (that is, in the making and reinforcing of social norms), I am not taking a strong stance on Buddhism so much as noting its effects, particularly when its premises are solidified as ontological givens and thereby put to use in social and political realms. Pity has come to signal an appropriate elevation of status that is needed in order to provide for another in Thailand. It is thus part and parcel of the patronage system, and shows us how linked such a system is to Buddhist doctrine and felt personal well-being as well.

Patronage

Somkiati is a former community health doctor turned high-ranking government official. One afternoon, after a morning packed with meetings with Chiang Mai University's medical faculty, a friend and I drove him to the airport for his flight back to Bangkok. Traffic was heavy, and what began as small talk soon developed into a more serious discussion. With decades of experience, Somkiati offered insightful reflections on the changes he has witnessed in health-care practice in communities across Thailand. He was for years a hands-on practitioner; he now travels the country as a senior official in the public health ministry. Unlike so many high-ranking officials, he recognizes the rote daily grind of intimate physical care and the inability of many professionals to acknowledge the know-how of those who do the day-in-and-day-out work. Thus his angle on health-care development—both in terms of professional and volunteer care—not only provides an overview of the structures of care, but also resonates with the experience of caregivers in my research in homes in Chiang Mai.

We began talking about the "rights" focus found in caregiving environments these days. A Patient's Bill of Rights was ushered in as part of the 1997 Constitution, transforming the legal framework of care, particularly in hospitals. It is a ten-point statement asserting basic entitlements—from the right to medical services regardless of status or identity, to the right to second opinions on treatment courses and full access to medical records.[25] The Bill of Rights is now prominently displayed in nearly every room of all hospitals throughout Thailand. Somkiati sees largely negative effects as a result. In his opinion, the formal arrangements enforced by such a rights-based approach have affected doctor-patient relationships. Whereas in the past doctors would do things for patients because they felt sympathy for them, now they are overworked and stressed and, in the face of patients proclaiming their right to care, they take a stand for their rights as doctors *not* to do certain tasks.

Recall Brapin's notion that it is necessary for a volunteer to feel pity (*songsān*, สงสาร) to help another in need. Somkiati agrees that care requires what he calls in English "sympathy": a term, as he uses it, akin to the Thai word for pity, perhaps combined with a degree of understanding (*khao jai*, เข้าใจ). Somkiati went on to say he felt that, rather than creating a more egalitarian system, the rights approach has made hierarchy "worse." Patient perspectives are increasingly ignored, as medical training emphasizes technological interventions, and rising opportunity costs make physicians shun community work in favor of higher-paying jobs in cities. In essence, Somkiati sees evidence of the breakdown of what he calls the "Thai patronage culture."

Implicit in the "patronage" view is the idea that with greater social status comes an increasing capacity to care for others. In terms of the social body, one might say this is akin to "heads" being able to keep the best interests of their "bodies" at the forefront; with the breakdown of this system, participation in collectives is a forced exercise of formal hierarchy rather than shared health maintenance. One can, and should, understand this as a conservative view of Thai society.[26] But the notion that the "pitiable" have some recourse to the patron system has deep and pervasive roots. The political is intertwined with the social and the religious; in turn, there are philosophical as well as practical barriers to casting off the paternalistic elements of this system.

The success of the Aw Saw Maw's long-standing public health volunteer system was, for Somkiati, a case in point: he saw forms of patronage as essential to the program's success. The program gives volunteers a connection with the government, which he said gives them a "little social boost."[27] Of all the volunteer groups in the country, Somkiati felt Aw Saw Maw conveys the greatest status. Somkiati could cite many people who claimed great benefits from the program, including village headmen and district leaders who rose from the ranks of Aw Saw Maw. And while my research suggests a mixed reception for volunteers at present, certainly as the program has developed into an institution, the system itself has the capacity to create status markers within its organization, and responsibilities and benefits increasingly flow therein. There is now a chief at every district level who has direct contact with chief medical officers and is often chosen as the provincial representative to travel to conferences and so forth. Again, with these benefits comes increasing ability to care for others. Somkiati felt the recent shift in policy to pay the Aw Saw Maw volunteers was the direct result of higher-ranked Aw Saw Maw members securing enough political clout to lobby the government for funding for themselves and their lower-ranked fellow volunteers.

Aom and Ying, too, offer a perspective on patronage. After two years hunching over their mother's air mattress, only about one foot off the ground on a plywood base, they got a new bed. It was a hospital bed, with easily adjustable sides and enough lift to bring their mother's body up to chest height. No more backbreaking bending. The difference was life-changing. Such a bed was prohibitively expensive for the family, but because they were not completely destitute, the aid organizations in Chiang Mai did not find them sufficiently in need for such a donation. Finally, they had an idea. Aom claimed it came to her while watching an episode of *Circle of Life*. If people so readily donate to those in need, why not appeal to a rich person to help with their plight? She asked her brother to tell their story to a rich business associate in Bangkok. Within a week, they had their new bed. In this way, the role of the pitiable is appealing. Even when people understand the limits and unreliability of such a pattern, having some recourse to the patron system provides at least the potential of a safety net.

As I recounted, the director of OPO confirmed there is a "social norm" among Thais to donate to those who are pitiable. Katherine Bowie (1998) has also brought attention to the class stratification evident in merit-making in Northern Thailand. In turn, Bowie locates resistance to hegemonic order in merit-making, casting appeals to charity as a "weapon of the weak," a mechanism by which the poor can influence the behavior of the better-off. Indeed, almost daily, Ying would ask me if I thought she was pitiable (*nā songsān*, น่าสงสาร), an appeal for particular forms of support that I might offer her as a relatively rich foreigner. Now, again, it was the intention of OPO's director to fight against exactly such a norm. He wants volunteers to work *with* older people, rather than *for* those they find pitiable. Overall, I think this is an effort to eradicate class stratification, rather than an attempt to take away a mode of resistance. But this is why we need a rendering of the physical and emotional components of class in analysis, as well as a finer-grained understanding of the habituations of its structures. Given the social training of awareness that continually serves to reinforce hierarchical relations between people, along with an implicit theory of mind that serves to restrain certain modes of communication and a karmic framing of predestined social roles that can serve to legitimize inequity, the task of change is a formidable one. What motivations will arise? By what means? And in what system?

One day the director explained to me one of the hurdles they faced in elder empowerment as a fundamental problem of "networks" in Thailand. He took out a pad and wrote the Thai word *khrɨakhāi* (เครือข่าย), or network, drawing a line between the two words of this compound: *khrɨa* and *khāi*. *Khrɨa*, he explained, literally indicated a structure like a "bunch of bananas," and he drew four lines fanning out from a central point to represent the term.[28] *Khāi* means "net," which he said should mean there are connections between nodes—and he drew connections between the lines just drawn. But, he said, crossing out the diagram, this was not the case. Instead, each bunch of bananas led simply to another bunch. "Top-down" arrangements prevailed. It was care work without a net.

Elder Person Clubs were a prime example. The central government proclaimed that such clubs were to be arranged in all districts, and district leaders would themselves participate in regional organizations, with regional representatives taking part in national-level planning. The problem was that, among the older people themselves, say at the district level, there was no communication. The same could be said for volunteers in a variety of programs, Aw Saw Maw and Aw Paw Saw included. There was "no net." Thus, reciprocal ties and grassroots systems were not emerging; programs and relations alike went through central command.

Without a doubt, the overall dominance of centralized control is manifest when those above are held as most appropriate for providing for those below. Still, care is enacted through these patronage structures and hierarchical relations. Many people find some solace by participating in a harmonious system, regardless of whether there is active control from the bottom ranks. The stakes of change are high. And yet people are clearly capable of different forms of interdependence. The Abhidhammic theory of mind presented in chapter 2, in fact, asserts the profound influence between people, and social behaviors in groups reflect subtle attention to others in myriad ways.

Indeed, change is occurring. As noted in the introduction, Thailand now has a universal health-care system, complete with the Patient's Bill of Rights and hospital accreditation procedures that enforce new patterns of patient communication. Patients and doctors are, it might seem, increasingly placed on more equal footing. No longer can we liken the patient to a supplicant seeking the aid of a doctor patron. Yet not everyone is supporting such changes. Somkiati's reservations about the new system reveal some unintended consequences of rights-based reform. Volunteers like Brapin, with their emphasis on pity, seem to choose the patron role; for caregivers and care receivers, roles emerge that "make sense" in familiar religious and social terms. Are the changes afoot indicating fundamental changes in the nature of the social body? And if so, how might care be enacted in new forms?

The "Genius" Body and the Specter of a Multiheaded Monster

Boonsii is a volunteer for OPO. We met many times over the course of my work with the organization, as she was an active player in the group's efforts to provide home-based care for older people in the Chiang Mai municipal area. Meeting with her early one morning, I quickly realized that this particular interview with Boonsii would be a semipublic affair. I could see a group had already gathered inside, as she led me up the stairs of the concrete slab hut that served as her community group's meeting place and bakeshop. I had planned for a rich conversation on caring in community; what I also got was a lesson on politics in an urban village.

A born activist, Boonsii had a master's degree in social science and was a clear leader in her small slum village in Chiang Mai city. It was a linear community, with dwellings built in a line along the remains of an ancient outer wall of the old Lanna capital. As city planners began to eye the wall for possible restoration as a tourist attraction, the community faced increasing threat of eviction, and Boonsii was tireless in her efforts to make a case for their rightful occupation (and in some cases, ownership) of the land. The small hut where we seated ourselves, among a group of several other "eldercare volunteers," was a prime example of such efforts: there an engaged group produced branded local products, including baked goods and artisanal crafts, for sale in the popular walking street markets in town. This was an "income generating project," also supported by OPO; it served not only to help the community's older people sustain themselves, but also as an opportunity to cast the community members as traditional Thais with inherent cultural value.[29]

Boonsii and I sat across from each other near the open-air window. To my left sat Serm, a quiet older man around eighty years old who took a low profile in community affairs but was often present and supportive from the sidelines. To Boonsii's right sat Adele, a stout woman in her mid-seventies who was particularly active as a volunteer for older people in the community. And on the floor sat Madge, a poised middle-aged woman who ran the bakeshop. Boonsii herself was only fifty-seven, but took her place as a village elder and leader among volunteers for older people, among other projects. That I, a foreign researcher, was singling her out for a formal interview added an extra boost to her status in the room, and I dutifully took on my role with all the corresponding postures of respect and deference expected.

We covered many topics over the course of nearly three hours together that morning. She talked about her mother and her family history, the death of her father, the birth of her children. She told me the story of her divorce, and how that heartbreak led her to practice meditation and fight for the betterment of women's lives in general. We discussed the four volunteer groups with which she worked for the rights of women, elders, children, and the poor. She talked of the plight of the older people she visited regularly, and Serm and Adele joined in with their own experiences. Boonsii echoed what were by then familiar NGO themes, including the importance of working with and through local groups and the need for trust among participants. Everyone seemed to agree, just as everyone seemed to join in her passionate response to the mounting pressures on their community. Boonsii appeared in many ways like a voice for grassroots organizing, a champion of the poor and the underserved. But her position in the larger frame of current events became clearer as our discussion ventured into the unchartered waters of Thai politics.

It was August 2009. The Yellow Shirts (the pro-royalist People's Alliance for Democracy, or PAD) had taken over the international airport in Bangkok nearly a year earlier in an attempt to force the government's hand to purge former Prime Minster Thaksin's influence in politics. The incident elicited the scorn of many Thais for the negative economic consequences and national embarrassment it caused and, particularly in the pro-Red north, the lack of repercussions its schemers faced. In the intervening months, the Red Shirt protesters (from the United Front for Democracy Against Dictatorship, or UDD), had proven their steady support among the countries' poorest regions, despite violent state repression that had hit a fever pitch in April 2009, just a few months prior. (Of course, more violence was soon to come. The events of April 2009 would pale in comparison to the brutal scenes reported from Bangkok in May 2010.)

Although outside observers tend to resonate with democratic ideals and to associate calls for increased participatory action with nongovernmental organization work, NGO affiliation does not necessarily predict political allegiance in this Thai mix. Many of the educated grassroots activists I spoke with refused to take sides, claiming a middle ground that rose above the power politics saturating both Red and Yellow movements. However, some NGO leaders, particularly those of the collaborationist bent (see chapter 4) with international affiliations, were long-standing Democrats and remained both disgusted with Thaksin and committed to obliterating Red influence in politics, even at the expense of media freedoms and voter-determined political representation. Admittedly, I was taken aback by this stance at first. I had been primed to associate NGO work around the world with participatory action politics, assuming that such ideals would predominate among the staff in this sector.[30] I came, however, to understand that there was a widespread presumption, even among some of those working most stridently for the rights of the poor, that Red Shirt supporters had been "brainwashed" as a result of their poor education; in turn, it was only through paternalistic reeducation and control of media sources that the country could get back on track.[31]

Nevertheless, many of the field workers on the ground in Chiang Mai had Red Shirt sympathies, and I found many Red Shirt supporters among the eldercare volunteers with whom I worked most closely. I knew, for instance, that Adele was a member of the Chiang Mai 51, a vocal and aggressive Red Shirt coalition in town. But it became apparent in our small group that morning that Boonsii was not of like mind.

Boonsii sparked things off by saying that grassroots organizers were against Red-Yellow divisions. She felt that these sides were selfish and left the most vulnerable groups to suffer the most. She claimed there was no quality or clarity in the leadership, and they "want[ed] to make gray in the land" with color-coded politics that strive to "change the rules" of the political game. I began to feel some bristling when Boonsii went on to claim that people do not understand the way things work, and that they follow Thaksin because of his use of the media as a power weapon. Adele began to counter with examples of media outlets that do not speak of or for Thaksin, but a back and forth was soon cut short. Madge, from her position on the floor, simply suggested quietly that if we talked too much, it would certainly get too hot in the small room. And with that reprimand, Adele pushed back ever so slightly from the table. She sat, upright but silent, for the remainder of our strained conversation. Boonsii retook the reins, and held court, so to speak, free now to voice her opinions without interruption. I noted Adele's legs shaking a bit, and once we had spent an appropriate amount of time on less controversial topics (including the delicious quality of their baked goods), the meeting disbanded.

In some ways, this encounter illustrates the functioning of the social body I argued for in chapter 3. Subtle cues were taken regarding the designated leader of the assembly, and steps were taken to ensure the group kept together. "Technologies of restraint" were deployed, following the common logic of psychosocial support, detailed in chapter 2, that encourages equanimity in the face of turmoil. But Adele's bristling may very well represent a new role in social relations. The Red Shirt movement may be providing a model for people to voice their complaints, whereas previously they may have held silent.[32] Does this indicate that the "genius" body is changing shape? That is, is hierarchy abating, opening more room for voice and leadership from previously lower ranks?

Urgent calls for "unity" coming from Central Bangkok certainly lent support to the notion that changes were afoot. In August 2011, the following headline appeared in the English-language newspaper, the *Bangkok Post*: "Ruling Democrats Urge Public to Observe King's Concerns for Unity."[33] The column recounts "His

Majesty King Bhumibol Adulyadej's concerns regarding the lack of unity and co-operation in society," and the then-ruling Democrat Party's hopes to use the parliament as a means to increase solidarity and squelch "undesirable movements" in the country.[34] Chief of course among their complaints were the UDD Red Shirts' actions, including a plan for supporters to dress in black on the upcoming birthday of Privy Council president General Prem Tinsulanonda and the circulation of a petition to impeach Prime Minister Abhisit Vejjajiva.[35]

Also in August 2011, Her Majesty the Queen created a slogan for National Mother's Day (her birthday, August 12), on the theme of unity:

> *Thai national anthem reminds Thais, day and night*
> *To always remember that*
> *For Thailand to continue to exist*
> *Thais must adhere to unity.*[36]

The exact wording for unity here is *sāmakkī* (สามัคคี), which can also be translated as harmony or community spirit. It comes as yet another reminder that Thais are meant to "love" harmony and unity; and in order to care for the nation, people must play their particular role as part of a larger whole. Of course, my argument for the social body is in phenomenological terms: people train their awareness on group dynamics through repeated embodied actions responding to social cues. What are we to make of these overt dictates, these explicit calls for unity? Unlike most readings, I think these should be considered as both strong-armed efforts to impose hegemonic social order and as expressions of care for the nation, however manipulative, through the maintenance of the status quo. For if one fails to consider the latter, it could lead to a similar failure to appreciate that some attempts claiming full revolution may merely seek an exchange of one ruling "head" for another.

By no means can one claim that lower classes have been aligned in calling for a different set of social roles. The majority of PAD supporters were fabled to be among the middle and upper classes, but one could not assume based on class where someone's political affiliations stood. I worked with many people living in extreme poverty who agreed wholeheartedly with Yellow Shirt–aligned television programming and warned me repeatedly of the dangers of venturing too close to the Red Shirts and their protest sites. A main aspect of this political turmoil in Thailand was a struggle not between rich and poor, but rather between elites.[37] Many seemed to support a reliance on old forms, simply with a new "head" on the hierarchical social body; to others, the fight for a new caste of leadership viscerally evoked what might be called, using the terms I have laid out, a grotesque social body with multiple heads.

When Prime Minister Yingluck Shinawatra was elected in August 2011, she was not what the royally aligned elite had in mind to re-instill unity. The first female prime minister in Thai history, she was also the sister of ousted Prime Minister Thaksin Shinawatra, and her party, Puea Thai, explicitly claimed to be the voice of the former PM. There was great tension before Yingluck's confirmation, as supporters worried that a judicial ruling would declare the election invalid. Opponents, on the other hand, thought all Shinawatras and their cronies claimed more "face" than they deserved. Having taken the helm from those who should rightly rule, Shinawatras threatened to morph the "genius of Thai society" into a hydra-headed monster.[38] Red Shirts, in turn, trumpeted a new distribution of resources, with schemes for economic development in poor rural areas. Again, some viewed this as the mere promotion of increased consumption patterns; others saw instead the emergence of emancipatory political engagement. The PAD Yellow Shirts clearly saw the former, and proposed a "New Politics" system, in which 70 percent of officials would be appointed rather than elected, following the logic that those who are so positioned in the social body should continue to determine society's moves. And such is clearly the case in the current ruling military government, which seized control of the country in May 2014 in a coup d'état. Under the banner of the National Council for Peace and Order, the military has taken on the power to name the prime minister and control various ministerial positions. In a referendum in August 2016, a military-based constitution was approved by popular vote (however fraught), complete with the transformation of key elected positions to political appointments. And with the passing of King Bhumibol and a continued escalation of lèse majesté charges, the military, at the time of writing (2018), appears to be fully committed to maintaining leadership. Christine Gray suggests too that we can look to the performance of royal *kathin* rituals to mark the re-creation of rank and confirmation of leadership through succession (Gray 2016)—reminding us to pay attention to the economic as well as social ties that create the hierarchy.

If it is so clear that the ruling elite seek the status quo, with the continued dominance of the few over the many, what of the main opposition? Are we to see "political resistance to royalist hegemony" in Red Shirts and subsequent anti-junta activism (Glassman 2011, 36)? Many analysts, including geographer Jim Glassman, certainly do. He traces how the development of capitalism was intertwined with the rise of this "royalist hegemony"—and he cites the fall of the Communist Party of Thailand in the 1970s as a moment when social cohesion fused with the royally led capitalist transformation of the countryside. For Glassman, it is the uneven development (inevitably) produced by deepening capitalist development that is breaking the system—as if, in terms of the social body, various parts are too polarized now, the roles of the poor and of the rich too far apart, to function under the auspices of a united whole. Thus, in the opposition, we are to find a rejection of hierarchical dominance, tout court. But Glassman also draws attention to the struggle not only between rich and poor, but also among elites—with various royalist networks on one end, and a variety of business and provincial power-brokers on the other. That the majority of the rural poor have chosen business and provincial powers by way of a Thaksin-inspired vision of economic prosperity, seems clear enough. But where Glassman sees a complete cracking of the overall social system, it is possible that familiar forms of attention to and care for the social body remain intact. Differential positions remain in society. Given the ways in which people find well-being in harmonious relations, many, at some felt level, may still welcome clear differentiation. Brapin certainly enjoys her ability to pity and patronize. The Red Shirts may deploy the rhetoric of egalitarian democratic ideals, but are its supporters merely demanding a leadership change? Are expectations of leaders changing? Is the entire differential structure shifting? As it should be clear, I think the mundane offers important clues to help answer such questions.

Changes Afoot and Footholds for Change

The rendering of different ways of being in the world found in this chapter and in this book as a whole, complete with historical trajectories and internal debate, urges a reconsideration of the relationships among state propaganda, religious ideology, and lived experience. Indeed, the vantage point of care shows clearly the imperialism of theoretical analyses that are not sensitive to the mutually constitutive effects of all three together. Take state propaganda: The prime minister's office invests an enormous amount in media advertising.[39] State budgets for popular programming suggest a presumed connection on the part of the state between viewing habits and political inclinations, but the blatant attempt at hegemonic dominance is but one element at play. This state propaganda does not operate in a vacuum; it emerges in a social context in which a long tradition has held that following prescribed means for maintaining harmonious social cohesion is the mode by which people best proceed toward living a good life. People feel themselves upheld by the collective. Granted, Gramsci defined hegemony in terms of the internalization of dominant ideas and people acting against their own self-interest; but we can be too easily relegated to decrying false consciousness without an appreciation of the embodied relevance and ulterior purposes those ideas can and do serve. In Thailand, from what vantage point can one unhesitatingly decry structural violence? Even taking a seemingly high road in advocating for compassion or empowerment or grassroots participation may inadvertently propagate power differentials between individuals and within small groups, which function in turn to maintain the status quo writ large.

Some promoters of volunteer activities see volunteerism as a means by which people can engage in religious action via physical, instrumental support of others. This is in some ways a "sincere" casting of action: the act itself is the object, and people are to bring their attention to it as such. For the director of OPO, this is meant to be a meeting of equals, a humanitarian-inspired endeavor of elder empowerment. For the Smart Merit campaign, the merit of prosocial action is a boon to one's community and one's spiritual development. But other volunteer activities are more rooted in the presumption that ritual action is of great benefit, with the ultimate object found in the plane of karma and merit, with emotional and social boons merely a symptom of a greater whole. So, for many of the people with whom I worked, what matters most—including caring for others, performing meritorious acts, and maintaining harmony in the social world as a means to both—is most easily pursued following well-worn performative ritual paths and social dictates.

Very often, when people see structural violence with clarity they feel driven to change the conditions in which people are suffering. A common implicit hope is that social analysis will be a mirror onto situations, prompting people to work toward ameliorating or obliterating patterns of domination. Here I have argued that within those very patterns of domination are the means and mechanisms by which people are providing for one another. And not only are they caring for one another in these ways, they are feeling cared for, as perverse as that may seem, through processes that maintain inequity and oppression. Thus one must bear witness to care, lest righteous calls for social justice commit another set of violences—failing to recognize the care people show for their world, stripping them of familiar forms of providing for one another, victimizing them through proclamations of false consciousness, and denying any creative possibility to use old forms in new ways.

Perhaps then the way to work toward the alleviation of disenfranchisement and systematic oppression is to offer care—that is, to understand what counts in context as providing for others and to pursue new equivalents in practice that achieve similar ends. How to do so I cannot simply announce; that seems to me the work of emergent processes, though in the conclusion I will offer notes on ritual in relation to change at individual, interpersonal, and organizational levels.

ON UNENDING CARE: RITUALS FOR MAKING THINGS SO

As we shuttled his mother to her monthly appointment at the hospital, Jidtuporn recounted key events of his life. He spoke of recklessly pursuing his first love, without paying heed to the consequences. Alluding to (but not detailing) his struggles, he related how his father thought he was losing his mind and convinced him to change his ways. Jidtuporn entered the monkhood for a time, which, he reported, changed his perspective and straightened him out. Decades later, he remained a sweet and gentle man, humble and devout, the epitome of the Buddhist layman. Jidtuporn himself did not claim such a status, of course. But his family understood him to be the most responsible and morally upright of Tatsanii's children. And he in turn reflected back to them an ethical frame for their family care situation: namely, that everyone helped according to his or her ability, with each role likely reflective of their respective karmic conditions. Since he had to work, his primary mode of support was through money and the monthly transport; two of his sisters, given their life circumstances, could physically tend to their mother at home, making a great deal of merit in the process.

Jidtuporn's biography mirrors a Jataka tale. First, like many of these stories of the Buddha's former lives, a morally questionable act readies the protagonist for teachings. A particular type of intersubjectivity is evident, as characters recognize their own moral status through the reflections of others. And, crucially, those with a sufficient degree of religious attainment are understood to see cause and effect more clearly than others, across time and space continuums, and thus able to decipher situations properly. In Jidtuporn's story, his father reflects his internal predicament back to him, prompting his ordination. And when Tatsanii is no longer able to care for herself, Jidtuporn is able to frame his family's circumstances and encourage them accordingly.

Framing caregiving situations is rife with pitfalls. What counts as providing for others in context is contingent on myriad factors, and what is justified at one level of analysis is often contradicted at another. But what people routinely do and how they are habituated to do it reveal a great deal about care and about the social world in which it occurs.

Jidtuporn's framing—that which he reflects back to his family as well as how they understand him—also arises in habituated forms. From personal narratives like Jidtuporn's (or that of Mam and others in chapter 2) to popular programming like *Real Life Dramas 84000* (as described in chapter 5), the basic forms of the Jataka tales find expression throughout contemporary Thai society. These narrative patterns are legible and convey meaning, along with whatever content the story recounts.[1] And, as I have noted, this patterning encourages an expanded time frame of analysis, a way of looking beyond immediate circumstances to less proximate causes of action, through the idiom of karma.

In this way, karmic reasoning resonates with efforts to identify structural violence. Indeed, some modernist renderings of karma mirror such analytical assessments of the systematic forces constraining individual and group behavior. For instance, Thich Nhat Hanh, a key figure in the Engaged Buddhist movement, stresses social circumstances as the cause of misfortune over and above individual karmic retribution.[2] He thereby justifies analysis of structural violence in and through basic tenets of karma. I am sympathetic to such analyses, though not completely satisfied with the approach. In part this is due to the perils of taking recourse in a religious framework. Granted, I too have utilized what can be characterized as a Buddhist philosophy through Buddhaghosa to help decipher the social landscape, particularly in relation to an operative theory of mind, and I have sought to identify Theravadin narrative forms and logics operating in the social world. But I have also documented the ways Buddhist tenets are mobilized in Thailand as justification for social oppression and political maneuverings, particularly throughout the later chapters of this book.

People inherit meanings through social practice, as when personal misfortune and social stratification are considered karmic indicators. Problematic meanings are all too easily reinforced. I have tried to interrogate such associations in previous chapters—from anger broadcasting one's karmic burdens (chapter 2) to gender-based social discrimination attributed to the repercussions of individuals' past actions (chapter 5). These meanings are not merely held in propositional commitments; they often have felt perceptual coordinates. People can become physically uncomfortable when prestige-bound rules of comportment are transgressed (chapter 3); and people give and find comfort in merit-making traditions, even in the face of other unmet needs (chapters 1 and 4). What's more, competing ideological stances on, for instance, the more supernatural elements of karma and merit have serious political implications (as interrogated in chapter 4), with no easy one-size-fits-all fix.

Thus, in the Thai cases I am describing, familiar forms of structural analysis are necessary, yet insufficient, for making sense of the contemporary moment and influencing the trajectory of social changes under way, from the demographic to the political. Examination of habituated action can provide a needed platform for interrupting harmful associations with calibrated alternatives, taking into consideration not just doctrinal stances but all that is embodied in routines as well. The remarkable thing that close attention to the caregivers I met in Thailand reveals is the way that what might otherwise be construed as merely political ideology (and thus located in the realm of ideas and discourse) is found in ordinary embodied experience. Take social harmony, for example. Military strategists, politicians, and conservative scholars alike can be found in Thai history to expound on something akin to what I have here called the social body. But while rhetoric that equates society with a body (from figures like Kukrit Pramoj in the twentieth century, for example) may seem a thin attempt to corral people into the party line of unity, I have shown embodied ways of being that continually habituate people into such a perspective. Beyond mere rhetoric, socially emphasized perceptual coordinates train people into such ways of being and knowing the world. We cannot, as effective scholars or activists, simply decry political strategies and ideologies as abhorrently oppressive or as instantiations of structural violence without taking into account the way people are complicit with and reliant on these coordinates in their everyday practices of care.

A focus on care in the pages of this book fosters the thick ethnographic description called for by Clifford Geertz, and echoed more recently by J. K. Gibson-Graham in service of revolutionary aims. As Gibson-Graham write, "Many ethnographic studies are focused on situations in which social relations are changing. . . . And in 'reading' change, it is difficult to resist the influence of 'strong theory'—that is, powerful discourses that organize events into understandable and seemingly predictable trajectories" (Gibson-Graham 2014). In turn, Gibson-Graham call for thick description and "weak theory" to enact noncapitalist realities. Structural violence arguably works at times as strong theory in medical anthropology, closing off alternative possibilities.[3] Nonetheless, many anthropologists who use the term aspire for their analyses to help make a better world, and many strive to keep alternative realities and social potentialities in view. I contend that open ethnographic engagement with care helps illuminate relationality and mutual aid amid hierarchy and tyranny and lays bare the needs and desires that yearn for fulfillment along any path to liberation.

Caregivers provide important insight into the necessary dynamics of sustained social change. In particular, the habituated means of providing for others, and the embodied forms by which perceptions are trained and care is enacted, underscores the types of transformations needed to support lasting alterations of the status quo at individual and group levels. In articulating the connection between social change and transformations in habituated action, I am inspired by the work of activists writing about and from within radical movements tuned in to somatics and emergence. By radical, I follow the meaning provided by Angela Davis: "Radical simply means 'grasping things at the root.'"[4] At root here is the training of perceptual awareness and embodied form, understood as inseparable from ideological commitments and visions of the future. The California-based group called "generative somatics" articulates something similar in its mission statement, seeking to grow a movement that "integrates personal and social transformation, creates compelling alternatives to the status quo and embodies the creativity and life affirming actions we need to forward systemic change."[5] Embodied actions are here inseparable from political analyses and a theory of systemic change. Rev. angel Kyodo williams, with colleagues (2016), claims a similar notion of "transformative social change," which she sees as driven by individuals' experience with breaking from dominator culture: that is, personal recognition of the patterns instilled in one's own body and cognition and the surrounding society, and experience glimpsing and embodying something new. Nick Montgomery and carla bergman (2017) provide examples of ushering in such change in terms of "joyful militancy." And adrienne maree brown (2017) draws inspiration from biomimicry and science fiction to relate a vision of "emergent strategy" for such change work, also deeply committed to embodied forms as much as any ideological commitment. In all these examples, among others, the need to retrain routines and develop new forms of relationality—to self and other—is readily apparent. So it is in line with this visioning that I have thought about how the caregivers in this book can help engage ritual in service of social change theory and praxis.

Rather than providing a framework for understanding how things "really are," I argue that rituals of care show an alternative mechanism for making things so. Ritual in this sense is a subjunctive mode that brings the world into being through acting *as if* it were a particular way, rather than claiming it to be so (chapter 1). As proponents of "radical dharma" suggest, "th[e] ability to disrupt our programming and form new cognitive connections based on direct experience that then becomes embodied through repetition—practice—is one of human beings' greatest attributes" (williams et al. 2016, 204). Ancient Chinese ritual theory suggests something similar. Drawing on the *Records of Rites*, written between the fourth and second century BCE and becoming one of the Five Classics in the first century

BCE, Michael Puett claims classic ritual theory is "not theory in the way we usually tend to use the word. These are not theories that attempt to describe the nature of ritual or the nature of the world. They instead work precisely like the rituals themselves, but at a meta-level" (Puett 2014, 231). Reading rituals as ontological treatises, we "domesticate" them, flatten them.[6] Instead, one can find in ritual, as Puett proposes, serious contentions regarding ways of engaging in the world for the betterment of human life. Ultimately, I am interested in Thai forms of ritualized care less because they are Buddhist and more because they are rituals, and as such, these ritual acts of providing for others show how one can make and unmake worlds without relying on notions of depth, sincerity, or ontology.

Through rituals of care, one can take seriously ways of acting "as if" actions accomplish certain ends and provide for others in particular ways, as the caregivers in this book do, rather than judging such acts as solid assertions of how the world is or is taken to be. Rituals thus serve our "plodding through" mundane life, as a guide to ethical action that builds over time. Showing up and going through the motions is of utmost importance. This became clear at the bedside as Aom and Ying (chapter 1) acted as if their actions of cleaning, feeding, turning, prodding, and powdering transformed unseen karmic burdens and accrued merit. The English word *care* may prime us to wed intention and interiority to acts of providing for others, but the context and conditions I describe urge us to put such correlations on hold. What emerges is a powerful foil to the post-Reformation Christian hermeneutics of the self, which are deeply rooted in dominant ideas about care as well as ritual. It can then become clear why "going through the motions" can spark repulsion in some contexts, especially those in which ritual often implies a sense of inauthenticity or insincerity. As Susan Stryker (2006) points out, in Western contexts there is a strong positive moral valence to "depth" and a negative valence to "surface," particularly when surface does not authentically map onto inner depths. Perhaps it is time to consider the limitations that such associations put on people's capacity to change harmful social norms.

An Abhidhammic theory of mind urges an alternative understanding of self-formation more congruent with ritual, in the subjunctive sense that I am using it. As Jidtuporn explained on the ride home from a particularly harrowing visit to the hospital with his mother (chapter 2), Thai people often act "as if" high-arousal mental states are indicative of negative karma or are otherwise unhealthy, and ideally follow social prescriptions for distraction and other forms of restraint to aid one another in the cultivation of healthy internal states. This makes sense in relation to the philosophical treatises that describe the "mind" as a collection of component parts bundled together, with intention but one component thereof. The agency and "patiency" of any given moment of experience punctures the notion of a true and enduring self, an inner conviction or decision maker that can be uncovered or expressed through authentic action. Instead, the self is transitory, a function of conditioning. Hence the importance of setting up situations that move people toward liberation. Prescribed actions can help people refrain from negative entanglements, contribute to the conditioning of wholesome internal orientation, and possibly even create the preconditions for actions (of body, speech, and mind) that do not produce karma at all.

Such a logic is not spelled out in every individual case I review in this book: rituals of this kind of interpersonal care can be inherited by convention and tradition. Perhaps so too in new traditions. Alternative modes of interpersonal support, such as found in the Confronting Death Peacefully initiatives (chapter 2), may ultimately function in a ritual mode. New ways of sharing emotional strife at the end of life seem from one angle to indicate a modernist call for sincerity in social communication. But how these injunctions are taken up and spread will matter. They may become rituals of care that simply provide new patterns of interactions through which people act as if their relations are strengthened by new modes of intimacy. Perhaps such patterns will better interface with, for instance, biomedical infrastructure—allowing people to discuss and make decisions about new life-sustaining treatment options, the likes of which traditional communication patterns did not have to contend. Perhaps only time can tell.

Regardless of the existence or rise of sincere frames in Thailand, rituals of care are still apparent in people's perception of, and participation in, the social body, as described in chapter 3. Thinking of social relations in terms of ritual provides "space" for people to know, at some level, that certain leaders are not looking out for their best interests—even as they carry out rituals that suggest they support those leaders and the status quo. In fact, failing to acknowledge ritual engagement risks presuming a type of "authentic action" in all social relations, which can leave virtually no choice but to ascribe something like "false consciousness" to lower-status people who perform hierarchical behaviors. What I have tried to show instead is a kind of care felt in acting as if one is a part of a larger collective body, regardless of position therein. And while it is not always the case, there is often a degree of influence to be found in playing one's part, even if "inauthentically."

There are rituals of care in Thai civil society, too, that provide mechanisms for people to provide for one another through set patterns of action. Volunteers' merit-making, like that of Mau Fah (chapter 4), is a prime example. Although ritual acts may fall short of certain needs, the performance of such acts need not be stripped of all legitimation and potential. Indeed, doing so is itself a power play in Thailand with old roots. As seen throughout chapter 4, judgments on others' religious attainment and alignment has historically been used to broker status, whether through advancing oneself as educated and cosmopolitan by decrying certain forms of practice as "not real Buddhism" or alluding to understanding "truth beyond truth" to bolster one's public platform.[7] Understanding operations of power along culturally specific lines is therefore necessary for sophisticated analysis and can suggest opportunities for innovative interventions as well. Ritual may be one such opening. Speaking in terms of a generalized social science perspective, Puett suggests, "Indigenous theories might help us to break down some of our own assumptions about how theory operates and to develop new ways of thinking with and through frameworks that are more deliberate in their transformative work" (2014, 232). It is my contention that rituals of care can do just that.

Seeing clearly how care takes ritual shape in Thailand offers building blocks for individual, group, and societal transformation. In terms of rote repetition, the basic stuff of care, ritual shows us how humans create dispositions—right down to norms of perception—that brings forward a means of reorientation and change impossible to produce by rhetoric alone. Doing is necessary. Doing is transformative, even when repetitive.[8]

I have come to feel caregiving can unlock universals of human experience as well as that which is very particular indeed. No matter the register—whether one-on-one or as part of a collective—caregiving is a trained, habituated activity. Aom and Ying have their tasks mastered. The procedures that took hours upon hours to complete when they first became caregivers are now accomplished in a fraction of the time. They learned by doing, their bodies becoming attuned to what was most important based on experience, based on feedback from the environment. Their awareness is automated, and that makes their care expert.

The same habituation is true for caring on other levels. I have unpacked Thai social habitus to reveal certain trained sets of engagements. Providing for others at increasingly social levels entails perceptual and physical conditioning that is predicated on particular historical, religious, social, and political parameters. This includes class hierarchy and the influence of Buddhist cosmology in the political realm. People talk explicitly about caring for their society (*kāndūlæ sangkhom*, การดูแลสังคม); *how* they do this is based on the lineage of care I have traced in this book.

My analysis of rituals of care highlights debates within Thai society about the role of pity in service to others, whether karma plays out over moments or across lifetimes, and even whether harmony is a positive social value or an imposed form of rule. These debates "make sense" in context and reflect what matters most to people in how and why to provide for others. But that these debates are not the same the world over emphasizes again that there are particular coordinates to care that scholarship can and must unearth. These alternatives also indicate that those of us conditioned to understand care as contingent on intention may have something to learn from care as practiced in other places.

It is true that there is a structural violence inherent in a social system that elicits "care" in the form of harmonious social relationships predicated on unequal social roles. Reliance on eventual transformations of merit and karma, rather than, say, equal resource distribution, reinforces hierarchy and its negative repercussions. That is not what I am advocating. However, to argue that hierarchical caregiving relationships are thus inherently oppressive is similarly unsatisfactory. To do so would posit a radical individualism that ignores the moral, spiritual, and deeply human connections embodied in even the most arduous or imbalanced caregiving relationships. What's more, such a blunt depiction ignores the possibility for value in hierarchy as well as the compromises individuals make within any social system.

Similarly, it is not appropriate to claim that the intimate tasks of bedside caregiving are of the exact same sort as the acts of care shown to society as a whole. This would require either a radical conservatism or a functionalist argument that simply does not bear out in ethnographic detail. Awareness is trained through engagement with social rules and norms; even perceptual patterns are affected by such conditioning. And as people begin to feel and make meaning based on the coordinates of their actions, I have shown they are often complicit with the ties that bind them. As with Jidtuporn autobiographically mimicking the Jataka tales, directives from the social world and its traditions serve, explicitly and implicitly, as guidance for right action. But while I argue that even the most spontaneous tending of bodies is imbued with a type of training, that which matters most is nevertheless continually negotiated. Structures that bind are always, ultimately, changeable, emergent as they are from habituated actions.

It may seem there is no way out—for my argument, or from the work of care itself. Caregiving remains a practice that demands compromise, that binds people even as it sets them free. Even when people's imaginations try to get them out of the caregiving bind, inevitably the complexities of the lived social world throw up barriers, and death itself remains the harsh eventuality of even the best care. And yet, ritual may offer a way onward. It may, in fact, be precisely because there is no way out—no hope, as it were, of making everything all right—that we can find the true power in rituals of care. Acting as if actions can make and change the world for the better provides a logic, even in modern worlds, that can compel people just to show up. Care is there to do. And what we do matters.

Notes

INTRODUCTION

1. Maw, like many elder Thai women, is referred to by kin and strangers alike as Yāi or Khun Yāi, meaning maternal grandmother.

2. Boonyuang is Yāi Maw's only child, and she took on the responsibility of caring for her mother with a certain type of resignation. Boonyuang herself had had only one child as well. That daughter died tragically in her twenties, shortly after the birth of *her* only child. Boonyuang is now left widowed, with only one granddaughter, who lives with her father a short distance away. Boonyuang rides her bicycle across town every day to be with her granddaughter—perhaps in an attempt to dilute what she perceives as the father's negative influence, or perhaps simply for the young company. Thus when I would come to visit, I often found Grandma Maw locked up alone in the house; I was never quite sure whether she could register my "call" through the small window.

3. National aging policies drew on UN mandates and models from other countries, particularly from Scandinavia and Japan, countries recognized as leading the way in aging preparedness. As a Buddhist nation, Thailand was said to have spiritual resources from which to draw to support home and community care. And as an undercurrent to all was a notion of social change able to create the conditions in which elders are once again revered and engaged members of society.

4. The issue of population aging fell largely under the Ministry of Social Development and Human Security, rather than under the Ministry of Health. Such jurisdiction may be responsible in part for the broader range of social considerations that come into formal government renderings of eldercare as opposed to those in palliative care.

5. See Knodel and Bussarawan 2017; Knodel, Vipan, and Napaporn 2013.

6. See Aulino 2017; Sutthichai, Napaporn, and Jiraporn 2002. At the time of my primary research (2008–2009), Thailand had not yet achieved "aging society" status nationwide, though older people made up over 7 percent of the Chiang Mai population. At the time of writing, projections remain on track for the number of older people to surpass that of children under age fifteen by 2018.

7. For more comprehensive reviews, see Sokolovsky 2009; Hashimoto and Traphagan 2008.

8. See Greenberg and Muehlebach 2006; Lamb 2014.

9. OPO seeks to support poor older people in need, to inspire active aging and elder empowerment, and to encourage others not only to respect elders, but also to volunteer time and energy to their cause.

10. See Aulino et al. 2014 for an overview; see also Sopranzetti 2018.

11. Pasuk and Baker 1996, 2002; see also Sopranzetti 2013.

12. Thailand is one of the so-called Tiger Cub Economies, along with Indonesia, Malaysia, and the Philippines—the Southeast Asian nations following the same export-driven economic growth pattern as the Asian Tiger Economies of Hong Kong, Singapore, South Korea, and Taiwan.

13. See Pasuk and Baker 2004; Connors 2003; McCargo and Patthamānan 2005.

14. For more on the creation of universal health care, inaugurated as a "national pilot" in the first three months of Thaksin's premiership and pushed into law soon thereafter,

see Harris 2014a and b. For a more thorough overview of all five main policies—village debt moratorium, Village and Urban Community Revolving Fund (VUCF), the People's Bank, One Tambon [district], One Product (OTOP), and Universal Healthcare (UC)— implemented during this period, see Sopranzetti 2013; Pasuk and Baker 2004.

15. See Klima 2002; Supasawad 2008.

16. As Thaksin explained, "Capitalism has targets but no ideals, while socialism has ideals but no targets [therefore] we need to combine the best of each. . . . I'm applying socialism in the lower economy, and capitalism in the upper economy" (Pasuk and Baker 2004, 118).

17. Sopranzetti proposed that Thaksinomics represents a return to the ideas of Milton Friedman's mentor, Frederich Hayek (Sopranzetti 2013). Tracing debates from the 1940s and 1950s in the Mont Pelerin Society, Sopranzetti finds evidence of a strong state even in Friedman's own early writings, as well as in those of a host of other "founding fathers" of neoliberalism. Sopranzetti thus argues for Thailand as a "neoliberal welfare state," with welfare understood not in the Keynesian fashion of support for those who are not able-bodied participants in the economy (the young, the elders), but rather welfare as the support of the entrepreneurial class. Sopranzetti's term "regulated neoliberalism" resonates with what has elsewhere been called "compensatory neoliberalism," both helpful (see Kasian 2015, following Perry Anderson).

18. Thaksin's influence, even for his signature universal health-care program, is increasingly downplayed. Thaworn Sakunphanit and Worawet Suwanrada frame both Keynesian and entrepreneurial welfare schemes as an "egalitarian approach" to governance and date advocacy for both forms of populist programming back to the 1970s, quite separate from contemporary Red-Yellow party divisions. They write, "An egalitarian approach to providing equal access to necessary health and social services was debated in the 1970s. Two decades later, after the economic crisis, social movements successfully managed to have the concept included in the 1997 Constitution, which led to a universal health-coverage policy in 2002. The efforts of other social movements and further advocacy by the organizations of the elderly pushed the idea of universal elder income security into the 2007 Constitution" (Thaworn and Worawet 2011, 412). There is no mention of Thaksin Shinawatra in the whole of the account. Although advocates of older person pension programs, like Thaworn and Worawet, downplay the influence of Thaksin in the success of these programs, political maneuverings are apparent. Abhisit's moves as head of the Democratic Party were seen by many Red Shirts as cheap attempts to superficially appease the poor. In turn, Democrats claim the government of Yingluck Shinawatra, Thaksin's sister, held up passage of the National Pension Fund Act because of party allegiances and increased payments under the universal pension as a means of claiming that program as its own. Party fault lines served to politicize certain schemes, though the will for state support became undeniable in the wake of a politicized electorate.

19. The Aw Paw Saw program is modeled after the highly successful and high profile Ministry of Public Health volunteer program, Aw Saw Maw (อสม), discussed in chapter 4. Currently over eight hundred thousand public health volunteers have a presence in every village, if not every family, in the nation. (For more details, see ลือชัย ศรีเงินยวง และ ยงยุทธ พงษ์ สุภาพ 2009.) Many other governmental bodies have since followed the volunteer suit, recruiting and using volunteers in nearly every ministry.

20. See Milligan and Conradson 2006; Ascoli and Ranci 2002. In the current literature, we find mainly European examples. As Marilyn Taylor notes, volunteer-based services are on the rise for adult care in the United Kingdom, but this generally represents a replacement of previously state-sponsored social services, as opposed to the inroads of state involvement that we see developing in Thailand (Taylor 2002, 91). It is helpful to remem-

ber that formal volunteerism generally includes provision of paid professionals who organize these volunteers, who themselves are increasingly called on to provide professional-level services but remain unpaid (or receive only marginal compensation). There is the possibility that volunteerism becomes a route to professionalization, as has been the case historically in other places, including the United States, though the trajectory remains unclear in this new neoliberal welfare landscape.

21. Muehlebach 2012 discusses the "production of compassion" for the poor and elderly in Italy, Rudnyckyj 2011 presents spiritual workshops in major state-run businesses in Indonesia, and Nguyen 2010 documents workshop strategies for producing "therapeutic citizenship" out of the AIDS crisis in West Africa.

22. Although infrastructure has been essential to instilling certain changes and trajectories in the colonial and postcolonial landscape, it often escapes and subverts capture in unexpected ways. Volunteerism thus proves a useful site of investigation in terms of infrastructure when the modes of engaging its content remain open for examination (see Wilson 2016).

23. Robert Desjarlais proposed "critical phenomenology" in *Shelter Blues* (1997), and I am similarly inspired to connect the phenomenal with the political, to trace how and why people do things, and to disrupt universalizing notions of agency. Where Desjarlais largely follows continental philosophers in that work, I will attempt to take major cues from Buddhaghosa and the Theravada philosophical tradition.

24. Husserl assessed that the "objective" or "true" world is, in fact, "a theoretical-logical substruction," and that "the objective is precisely never experienceable as itself" (Husserl 1970, 127 §34d). As a result, he decried a "crisis" in Western sciences, stemming from positivistic reduction that led to the very notion of mere fact and thus the loss of science's meaning for life.

25. See Bell 1997 for an insightful and synoptic review of ritual studies. My use of ritual, as detailed in chapter 1, most closely follows Seligman et al. (2008), who focus on the ways repetitive ritual acts create a *subjunctive*: a means by which people can act *as if* the world were a particular way, even without ultimately believing it to be so. Within this frame, a diverse set of activities qualify as ritual—from handshakes and polite greetings to baptisms and ordinations—in contrast to classic distinctions between the sacred and the profane, the religious and the technical, or the ritualized and nonritualized elements of a diverse set of actions (as in Leach 1954). What follows bears some resemblance to studies of ritual performance in the context of healing, in the sense of ritual as performance *doing something* in the world (see Laderman and Roseman 1996). Nevertheless, ritual here is not presumed a priori to be representational or even functional for the social world; rather I pay close attention to what is actually done (see Handelman 2005). Thai social worlds and the philosophical lineages most relevant to them encourage appreciation of habituating actions as a pattern of ritual (more than the details of any given rite) and an understanding that consequences may arise outside of this worldly space and time.

26. It might be argued that this is the dominant perspective in and out of academia. But there are of course important exceptions to this characterization, some discussed in chapter 1. Annemarie Mol (2008) and Mol and colleagues (2010) move against this grain with a decided focus on care in practice. But a centering question in my work is how to locate the patterning of value and experience within practice.

27. See Martin, Myers, and Viseu 2015 for a productive review, as well as the entire special issue that it introduces. See also Mol et al. 2010; Puig de la Bellacasa 2017; Tronto 1993.

28. This leads even seemingly universal or open frames to remain overdetermined. For instance, Michelle Murphy, in her work on "mobilizations of care" in feminist health practices and technoscience, writes,

Care carries (at least) four different interlaced meanings: first, it refers to the state of being emotionally attached to or fond of something; second, it means to provide for, look after, protect, sustain, and be responsible for something; third, it indicates attention and concern, to be careful, watchful, meticulous, and cautious; while its fourth meaning (and the first in the Oxford English Dictionary entry) is to be troubled worried, sorrowed, uneasy, and unsettled. (Murphy 2015, 721)

Based on my work in Thailand, I see many of these facets carry "baggage" from both the English language and philosophical lineages of the West. The Thai perspectives I present here unsettle common renderings of emotional attachment and expressions of concern, the locus of responsibility and the connotation of worry. Thus, again, I back up and define "care" more generically—simply as "providing for others"—to enable a more robust analytic category with clearer relevance cross-culturally, an opening for careful investigation at once "unsettling" and generative.

29. Here I build on anthropological expansion of the concept of "theory of mind." Developmental psychologists first coined the term "theory of mind" to refer to humans' ability to infer the thoughts or perspectives of others. While the root term is limited to a particular capacity for inference in the psychological literature, Tanya Luhrmann (2011) and other anthropologists recognize the implications of "cultural variations in models of mind inferred by social actors in different social settings" (5). Local theory of mind invites an appreciation of the logics by which people experience themselves, the world, and other people in it.

30. The very categories of the Pali Canon and Theravada Buddhism are not without their pitfalls, as many have noted (see Collins 2013); Heim (2014) goes a long way in moving through these tensions.

31. Perhaps it is a remnant of a misplaced hierarchy of value that so many scholars (anthropologists included) can seamlessly draw on Aristotle (384–322 BC), Augustine (354–430 AD), and Kant (1724–1804) to wrestle with contemporary theoretical concerns around the world, but rarely reach in the same way to Gautama Buddha (563–483 BC or 480–400 BC), Buddhaghosa (401–500 AD), or Ledi Sayadaw (1846–1923) as thinkers, philosophers, and theorists of the self and the social world.

32. It is worth noting that "mind" can be used in various ways, with varying degrees of specificity and/or concreteness, depending on the level of analysis deployed. In a similar fashion, certain adepts are thought able to discern the operations of karma across lifetimes; for others, acknowledgment of the general process suffices.

33. See Desjarlais 2003; Desjarlais and Throop 2011; Fassin 2012a; Kleinman 2006; Lambek 2010; Robbins 2007, 2009; Zigon 2008, 2009a, 2009b; cf. Mattingly 2014. Morality and ethics can be deployed in different ways, depending on the context or scholastic lineage. For example, Arthur Kleinman uses "ethics" to refer to an overarching code of right and wrong, and "morality" for the everyday instantiation of what matters most amid practical restrictions; other scholars use these terms in the inverse. Whether explicitly eliciting such a distinction or not, ethnographic focus tends to rest on extraordinary moments that are thought to lay bare underlying value schemes; following Foucault, this is understood as "a kind of reflective and reflexive stepping away from the embodied moral habitus or moral discourse" (Zigon 2008, 18), brought about by what Jarrett Zigon calls "moral breakdown" or problematization. I contend that habituated routines can reveal the local coordinates of the "moral basis of caregiving" (Kleinman 2007, 2008, 2009), not only highlighting how living a locally moral life can stand in tension with dominant ethical dictates, but also opening us up to the ambivalence, ambiguity, and potential malleability of the everyday practice of care.

34. See Blackman 2013 for more on the fascinating history of ideas surrounding habit, conscious choice, and the naturalization of the will.

35. As Paul Farmer defines the term, "Structural violence is one way of describing social arrangements that put individuals and populations in harm's way. . . . The arrangements are structural because they are embedded in the political and economic organization of our social world; they are violent because they cause injury to people. . . . Neither culture nor pure individual will is at fault; rather, historically given (and often economically driven) processes and forces conspire to constrain individual agency. Structural violence is visited upon all those whose social status denies them access to the fruits of scientific and social progress." (Quoted by Adam Burtle on http://www.structuralviolence.org /structural-violence/, accessed November 23, 2016.)

36. In their call for "alterpolitics," Ciavolella and Boni (2015) are committed to horizontal, as opposed to hierarchical, political formations. But clearly hierarchy must be considered in practice, not just ideology. As Nazima Kadir, speaking of her work in the squatters movement in Amsterdam, attests, "I have witnessed activists unwittingly reproducing and being embedded in the very social and cultural norms that they verbally reject" (Kadir 2016, x).

37. See Tausig 2013; Elinoff 2014.

1. THE KARMA OF CARE

1. The family and hospital staff referred to her state as "coma." This may, however, be a vernacular term, since there were indications that "persistent vegetative state" would have been more medically accurate. Nevertheless, Tatsanii's family always maintained the possibility that she could awaken.

2. As described in the introduction, the United Nations' definition of an "aging society" is one in which at least 7 percent of the population is over the age of sixty-five. In Thailand, 10 to 30 percent of older people require some aid in daily activities; of those who are unable to do at least one basic activity on their own, 40 percent of men and 65 percent of women are being cared for by a child or in-law, and about 3.5 percent of the elder population depends completely on full physical aid (Knodel and Napaporn 2009; NCE 2004). So while the intensity of care presented in this chapter is currently required by only a small percentage of older people, the axioms of practice found in this case are quite common, occurring all over Thailand and particularly in Chiang Mai, which has the second-largest population of older people in the country. Admittedly, the focus on "family caregiving" that emerges in this so-called aging crisis is subject to normative biases, and, as John Borneman (1997) has pointed out, "care" can and must trump "kinship." My attention here is on daughters as family caregivers, but the same patterns and ambivalences could be found in care provided by a host of others.

3. Outstanding examples include: Dole 2012; Garcia 2010; Han 2012; Kleinman 2009; Mol 2008; and Stevenson 2014.

4. See Povinelli 2011 for a discussion of the tendency to transform the mundane into an object of analytic concern or importance.

5. See for example Buch 2013; Hendriks 2012; Mol, Moser, and Pols 2010.

6. Elana Buch's (2015) article on aging and care highlights terrific examples of embodied practice in the literature, but as she attests, "ethnographic work focused on daily care practice is overwhelmingly based in European and North American contexts."

7. In a refreshing departure from common analytic blending of care in practice and care in reflection, Janelle Taylor powerfully acknowledges, "I am not the one who does most of the hard work of meeting my mother's practical needs" (2008, 323); through her experiences we can see the necessity of confronting both opportunities for ethical reflection

provided by care scenarios and the "hard work" of meeting "practical needs" day in and day out in different settings.

8. See Aulino 2014; Fassin 2012a; Lambek 2010; Mattingly 2014; Robbins 2007; Shohet 2013; Zigon 2009a and b.

9. Julie Livingston explains, "The moral philosophy of Batswana nurses, with its emphasis on empathy—on the ability to perceive another's suffering at the level of feeling, and to then in turn transform that suffering by recalibrating their own bodily consciousness—offers deep insights into the intersubjective phenomenology of care" (2012, 111–112). It is precisely here that we need to calibrate this insight to the Christian-inflected Botswanan context. At root, *bongaka* (Christian Botswanan therapeutics) assumes that bodies are permeable to the thoughts and feelings of others, providing a focal point for moral action. In contrast, in Thai Buddhist contexts in which I work, many people understand thoughts and feelings as necessarily fleeting. The corresponding moral code generally involves distracting others from their anguish, as discussed in chapter 2, which may circumvent the need or desire for the type of "recalibrating" transformations provided by nurses in Botswana. Understanding competing theories of interiority or mind, and their historical lineage, emerges as a crucial component of deciphering local conceptions and experiences of care.

10. It will become clear that this move is crucial for unearthing conceptions of the self that separate body, speech, and mind into distinctive factors with an extensive elaboration of the arising of and interdependence of each.

11. Rodney Needham (1972) cautioned against the unproblematic rendering of belief itself, but my argument does not merely rehash an old debate about whether certain internal states exist universally or whether the ethnographer can or cannot render internal states legible. Instead, I propose that attention to ritual challenges common (at times implicit) renderings of the internal correlates of care.

12. This discussion of Theravada Buddhist terminology is based on popular usage (see McDaniel 2011). Maria Heim (2014) offers the closest parallel interpretation of textual sources.

13. As Heim defines it, "karma means, at bottom, action, particularly action that is both the result of previous conditions and brings about future effects for the agent" (Heim 2014, 3).

14. There is an element of obligation here as well, reflected in the popular injunction to care for your parents as they cared for you as a babe. The need to repay such a debt reflects a sense of filial piety in the system of merit and karma. And, particularly for mothers, there is a promoted sense of the nearly godlike stature of one's mother.

15. See Sommai Premchit and Amphay Dore 1992. Ara Wilson (2004) contextualizes this logic in terms of a pervasive "folk economy" of transformative exchange. Men can repay their debt to their mothers by becoming monks, whereas women, restricted from ordination, participate in this logic of exchange by providing physical care.

16. This framing of ritual resonates with certain strains of performance theory—particularly that which stresses the material over the mental (even when trying to eliminate the false dichotomy between the two) and that which emphasizes the subject as the "product and process of repetition" (Morris 1995, 576).

17. The corresponding psychological correlates are explored in depth in chapter 2. There are indeed subjective clues to the results of actions or the "perlocutionary effects" of ritual actions; but feelings, their analysis, and appropriate modes of internal cultivation follow an Abhidhammic logic that demands extensive and separate renderings.

18. With the phrase "hidden in plain sight," I quote Aba Cecile McHardy from personal correspondence (see also Good 2010).

19. As noted above, Foucault (1988) provides a genealogy of this modern, liberal self, closely linked to a Christian hermeneutics of the self. The focus is on interiority and an

alignment between inner thoughts and feelings (which require scrutiny for proper ascertainment) and outward actions. There is an interesting corollary between this emphasis on interiority and what Peter Burke (1987) has called the historically situated "repudiation of ritual." As he asserts, "The Reformation was, among other things, a great debate, unparalleled in scale and intensity, about the meaning of ritual, its functions, and its proper forms," from which "ritual" emerged as "a bad word" (Burke 1987, 226 and 224). Luther and Calvin came to reject the efficacy of ritual acts without a corresponding belief—in contrast to medieval notions of ritual efficacy (*ex opere operato sine bono motu utentis*)—and radical Protestants like the Quakers even abandoned conventional greetings and other ritualized social engagement for their conceived artificiality (ibid., 228 and 233). This demand for "authenticity" has found its way into anthropological theory, as noted above and by Richard Handler (1986), who not only traces the western European construction of authenticity and its relationship with individualism, but also shows how it has crept into commonsense notions of culture. For studies of care, Handler's call is just as pressing as it was thirty years ago: "Our critical awareness of 'authenticity' will help us to bring new perspectives to bear on the study of others, and on ourselves studying others" (4).

20. The tendency to read "good care" as an index of certain internal states reproduces a type of scholarship born of Christian roots. Seligman and colleagues (2008) go so far as to posit that the modern world's predilection for absolutism and its desire for overarching coherence stems from a sincere frame that is particularly strong in fundamentalist movements. In deconstructing the concept of religion, Talal Asad finds that the quest for coherence is itself part of a Christian project and that a universal definition of religion is unattainable because it is "itself the historical product of discursive processes" (1993, 29). Webb Keane too notes the "normative ideal of sincerity"—whether specifically religious or otherwise elitist—in efforts to "reform the subject" into an autonomous, modern individual via Protestant conversion; further, Keane emphasizes how this ideal has become "part of the taken-for-granted background for the liberal tradition out of which have emerged many of the questions, methods, politics, and worries of anthropology and related disciplines at both the epistemic and ethical levels" (2002, 65). Drawing attention to rituals of care disturbs such tendencies. For questions of caregiving, it would be an error to leave these tendencies unchecked, lest an evangelical-type fervor sweep aspects of human experience out of view.

21. For more on the uses of ritual in the Thai context, see Morris 2002.

22. In Lionel Trilling's terms, "congruence between avowal and actual feeling," or "single-mindedness," is presumed in this sincere mode (1972, 2 and 111).

23. The differences in belief and practice patterns do not map neatly onto class and age categories, though modern discourse does dominate in elite rhetoric. See Ito 2012 and Wijeyewardene 1986 for insight into long-standing debates within Thai Buddhism. Nor does this firmly fit a necessarily Buddhist frame alone. Northern Thai metaphysics does not neatly map onto classic Buddhist texts or philosophy. In a cosmos that defies precise classification, Buddhism adds moral dimensions and personal responsibility to fate through the logic of karma: as Richard Davis explains, "The fortunes of individuals are unpredictable, but the forces affecting the course of one's life can be influenced by the correct application of ritual technology" (1984, 72).

24. I unpack the historically rooted assumptions and motivations at play in the deployment of such religious modes in Thailand as the book progresses. The trick is that key interpretations of the Pali texts are conceived in a modernist paradigm as well, thus rendering these texts in English using terms that pervert or otherwise "graft" Western thought onto Buddhist categories (see Heim 2014, 24, fn 57, with reference to McMahan).

25. Alan Klima argues that such elite discourse regarding Buddhism holds out "a difference that legitimates Euro-American values as quasi-universal . . . . Ironically, the source

for this Buddhist otherness is often, historically, an adoption by the purported 'others' of what they themselves perceived as either Western or modern styles of thinking" (2002, 19).

26. Although Seligman et al. (2008) suggest that modern societies "no longer have ritual as such a resource and must rely on . . . a sincerity mode of interaction as a mode of negotiating ambiguity" (46), I suggest instead that caregiving may after all be a contemporary form of ritual—even without the karmic coordinates—in other contexts as well.

27. My ethnography encounters Aom and Ying at a particular point in their caregiving experience, after years of performing a routine that has become ingrained in their daily affairs. I cannot speak to the role of conscious reflection in the learning of their tasks or their early framing of their care work. And while I hold fast to the emphasis on action over sincerity, this is not to say that intention or motivation does not change or otherwise come to bear on people's ethical reflections about their caregiving. The focus here is on moral practice and the proper characterization of the everyday.

28. In Thai, *rao mai dtông rïan trœsdï rao phãkptibat* (เราไม่ต้องเรียนทฤษฎี เราภาคปฏิบัติ); what I translate as "practice" can also be rendered as "field training."

29. This is reminiscent of Muehlebach's discussion of the Italian government: as it provides a normative account of volunteers that presumes their "affective and empathic stances," it fails to leave room for alternate orientations (2012, 104). What a pity if anthropological analyses were to do the same. Instead, a focus on care as providing for others can draw out these biopolitical maneuverings as they attempt to influence ways of assessing and meeting needs, and even underlying notions of the self.

2. THE CONDITIONING OF CARE

1. Writing of the Tibetan context, Lichter and Epstein claim, "The karmic value of an act depends largely upon the actor's intentions (*bsam-pa*, Sanskrit *cetana*)—as does merit gained by faith" (1983, 242).

2. Indeed, I presumed feelings would be a major component of both end-of-life and long-term care. I prepared to be receptive to the voicing of the fear, angst, guilt, sadness, or general emotional upheaval that I predicted would come with an adequate level of intimacy. And, having witnessed a great deal of such emotional sharing during my time as a hospice volunteer in the United States as well as in work on palliative care policy and programming, I suppose I fancied myself sensitive and trustworthy for such disclosures as well.

3. Sections or "chapters" of the booklet include 1. Who Is the Caregiver? 2. Your Feelings. 3. Asking for Help. 4. Caring for Yourself. 5. Going with Your Loved One to Medical Visits. 6. Talking with Others. 7. Remember. See http://www.cancer.gov/publications /patient-education/caring-for-the-caregiver.pdf.

4. Julia Cassaniti's work (2015) also challenges the presumption of emotional suppression.

5. Here I build on T. M. Luhrmann's anthropological theory of mind paradigm (2011), as described in the introduction to this book.

6. In his lectures in *Technologies of the Self*, Foucault traces a genealogy of practices related to self-examination and disclosure for personal cultivation, including practices in Greco-Roman philosophy (first and second centuries AD) and Christian monastic principles of the late Roman empire (fourth and fifth centuries). Foucault frames these strategies as one of four technologies with which humans understand themselves (including technologies of production, sign systems, power, and the self) and also as one of four parts of an analytical framework on ethics (composed of the substance of ethics, modes of subjectivation, techniques of the self, and telos). (See Foucault 1988. For extended discussion of Foucault's analytical framework on ethics, see Mahmood 2012.) Obedience and renunciation become prominent in Christian thought and practice through confessionals.

7. The title of this chapter, and much of its content, is indebted to Maria Heim's remarkable work (2014) bringing Buddhaghosa's ideas to light. Heim homes in on the abandoning, rather than the cultivation, of particular mental states in the Abhidhamma; and she turns to look at the Vinaya, the moral code of conduct for monks, as "a body of practical guidance on the technologies of restraint" (2014, 131).

8. Such an explanation was especially clear among a subset of middle-class, middle-aged women who frequently listen to sermons on tape and place a high importance on Buddhism in their lives. There are several fundamentalist Buddhist sects and smaller subsets of cosmopolitan Buddhist ventures throughout the country, as discussed in chapter 5, and to some degree this is common in their discourse as well.

9. The stakes in Thailand have always seemed high to me in this regard. Failure to think about and appropriately respond to the unstated needs of others is in some sense a failure of being Thai. In his influential monograph *Siam Mapped*, the Thai historian Thongchai Winichakul (1994) discusses the amorphous concept of Thai-ness, *khwām pen thai* (ความเป็นไทย), and the often-repeated accusation that foreigners can never really understand it. `*Ao jai khao mā sai jai rao* takes a similar form, in that everyone readily acknowledges its importance and claims its practice, but cannot necessarily define or describe the ways and means of its deployment. In the Western canon, I have found Edith Stein's 1917 treatise *On the Problem of Empathy* most related to the Thai concepts here, though the Pali Canon is more relevant in this context. Suffice to say, Stein casts empathy as the capacity to recognize others at all. So where her teacher, Husserl, took for granted that there were other "I's" (consciousness foreign to oneself), Stein asked how one knows that. She deduced in turn an innate empathic capacity rather than a sense constituted out of experience. I go on to show how the Abhidhamma lays out far greater nuance regarding this innate capacity than Stein was able to attain. (Sawicki 1998 provides a useful orientation to Stein's work in this regard.) What becomes of utmost importance in cultural analysis then is the trained focus on empathic recognition and the naturalized reactions of response.

10. Cassaniti emphasizes calmness as the result of letting go, an aim in itself; my sense is that calmness also has to do with facilitating accurate or otherwise appropriate sensory perception.

11. As Cassaniti reports, scholars have suggested that there may be two Buddhist "paths" at play here: one *kammic*, dependent on the accumulation of good merit, the other *nibbanic*, resting on the ideal of not accruing any karma (see Cassaniti 2015, 156n7). She shows how people reconcile the two, suggesting that "good new karma can be seen as practice in making no karma at all through emotional practice" (156). It is this idea that I hope to gain a more precise handle on.

12. Heim adds a fourth dimension to the standard parsing of the Pali Canon: narrative. Often categorized as part of the Suttas, the Jataka tales are stories that illustrate and develop the teachings in important ways.

13. In a similar fashion, the fact that Theravada texts are not spread uniformly, that they are taken up in different ways and expounded on variably across time and place, is itself an extension of the philosophy.

14. I am, of course, simplifying these philosophical tenets with a focus on karma—how could it be otherwise in such limited space? In classic Abhidhamma style, "*kiriya* is further clarified in a list of four types of intention that differs (but in certain overlapping ways) from the four dark and bright karmas. . . . The four types of intention are good (*kusala*), bad (*akusala*), resultant (*vipaka*), and *kiriya*" (Heim 2014, 64). As explored later, *arhats* are said to operate with no intention, the ideal for those seeking to escape suffering and the cycle of rebirth. Karma bears fruit, just as do five other elements—desire, feeling, perception, the depravities, and suffering—constituting the six "fundamental aspects of human experience . . . a somewhat expanded version of the five aggregates" (38). Heim is

concerned with intentionality, which is often directly equated with karma in the Canon (39), and I continue this focus on karma as it most directly relates to my experience in the field. Heim demonstrates how the stories of the Jataka tales (in another basket of the Tipitaka) flesh out the notion of the intersubjectivity that stems from this understanding of component parts—specifically how "Buddhaghosa acknowledges how our intentions are shaped by others in his exegesis on *cetanā*" (Heim 2014, 194)—which plays well with a focus on care too.

15. There are political ramifications for such a stance, which I discuss at length in chapter 5. The inaccessibility of non-karma-bearing intention to most people may lie behind Cassaniti's assertion that, for merit-making actions, "it is the intentional feeling that does the work" (2015, 98). But taking on intention in this way shortcuts the philosophical tenets at play.

16. "I believe that the language of absences is not just a quirk of the Pali but rather an important feature of this moral psychology that identifies experiences of absences as the conditions for other experiences that cannot otherwise occur" (Heim 2014, 79).

17. In the story of the woman and the monks, "The emotion that drove her action is not something located just in her head, but is in a complicated way tangled up with these particular monks; it exists *between* them." (Heim 2014, 194, emphasis original).

18. For example, consciousness in the technical rendering is but one of the five aggregates, one of four components of the fourfold nature of reality, with four planes of consciousness, and so forth in multiple divisions and combinations. In grosser accounts, a simple gloss of thinking or mind suffices.

19. In subsequent chapters, I further illustrate correlations between ancient and contemporary Theravada platforms, including popular television programming.

20. For more on nondisclosure of terminal prognoses in the Thai context, see Temsak Phungrassami et al. 2003; Stonington 2012, 2009.

21. As Heim argues, "While for Keown no English word matches *cetanā* precisely, he describes it as a type of practical reasoning or a kind of deliberation and decision about ends. But he also suggests that *cetanā* contains some dispositional and affective aspects. In fashioning his comparison with Aristotle, Keown wants to see the mind divided into the classic tripartite division of cognitive, affective, and conative elements, where the conative function, *cetanā*, 'is best pictured as the matrix in which the push and pull of the rational and emotional aspects of the psyche are funneled in the direction of moral choice'" (Heim 2014, 19, citing Keown 1992, *The Nature of Buddhist Ethics*, 216).

22. For similar arguments, see McMahan 2008 and Lopez 2002. McMahan argues for multiple modernities, including Asian modernities, playing out tendencies of modernity and showing how they arise differently across settings. But although different ages and contexts may bring different elements in this dynamic tradition to the fore (see also Schedneck 2015), dangers remain of misreading based on cultural biases.

23. Heim tracks the Christian moorings of these notions of the will from Saint Augustine, along with Protestant elaborations of "inner space" and conscience (see Heim 2014, 22–24).

24. In discussing this possibility, a trusted friend suggested the term *klan* (กลั้น) or *klan jai* (กลั้นใจ) as the relevant term. *Klan* has a meaning of holding or restraining, as in to hold one's breath. And indeed, the Royal Institute (1982 version, see http://www.thai-language.com/id/133145) defines the word in terms of "emotions" or "things which are inside the body" that are "forcibly or mandatorily unexpressed." There are of course times when such suppression of expression is impossible. A dictionary sample sentence describes such an instance: *lāi khrang thī thalǣngkān kānprachūan khǭng phra`ong mai sūdīnak lāi khon kǭ* **klan** *nāmtā wai mai yū* (หลายครั้งที่แถลงการณ์การประชวรของพระองค์ไม่สู้ดีนัก หลายคนก็กลั้นน้ำตาไว้ไม่อยู่), "On many occasions when the announcements regarding their health were not favor-

able, many people were *unable to* **hold back** their tears" (emphasis added). Though no one used this exact verbal formulation in interviews with me, the possibilities and even value of holding things inside is indeed evident in such a term.

25. There are Thai rituals for saying apologies right before death, such as the ritual to `ahōsikam* (อโหสิกรรม), which Bee has incorporated into her work. This involves cleansing the negative karmic effects of any wrongdoings and/or ill will between people. To have the opportunity to do this is thought to be a function of one's merit.

26. For comparative perspective, see Good et al. 1994.

27. See Gawande 2014 regarding the skill involved in breaking the news of a terminal prognosis.

28. See Good et al. 1994; Christakis 1999.

29. She also admitted she could not believe she was dying because she felt she was a good person, that she had merit, and that such a fate could not be hers—echoing common reactions documented at the end of life in Thailand (see Stonington 2009).

30. There are comparisons to make between the practices of care in Thailand and Japan. See Traphagan 2004; Long 2005.

31. See, for example, Good 1995.

32. A confluence of contemporary ideas are occurring in the Confronting Death Peacefully workshop, as in the "reflective" and "contemplative education" project the workshop is a part of. (See พระไพศาล วิสาโล 2549 [2006] and 2003; for network information, see http://www.budnet.org/sunset/; on changes to clinical subjectivity reflected in such activities, see Stonington 2011.) The explicit intention of the workshop is to open a space for personal reflection. But I am not alone in my critique of its heavy-handedness in this regard, as if organizers are attempting to lead people to specific reflections.

33. Of note, Heim calls attention to the "blunt" description of emotion in Buddhaghosa's work. This is not an elaborated or refined detailing of different emotional states, but basically a good, bad, neutral categorization—all that is necessary.

34. I describe in greater detail the processes involved in attending to groups in this manner in the next chapters. Of course, people find ways to subvert constraints on expression in both personal and political realms. Thus you have what Michael Herzfeld (2005) calls "social poetics" at play—where people communicate multiple meanings even through actions that on the surface follow social norms to a T. Ironic plays on words and gestures then allow for continual reconstitution of the ordinary.

35. These poems make up one of five parts of the Suttas, or teachings and sermons of the Buddha, which includes a mix of poetry among other writings. So, although less well known than the Jataka tales (verses about the Buddha's previous lives), these first poems of women Buddhists are along the same lines. But unlike the Jatakas, they are unique to the Theravada Canon; that is, they have no match or parallel in other Buddhist schools. Nevertheless, Hallisey indicates that they contain generic themes of Buddhism, along with a rendering of the social conditions of their time period. Rather than reading them for their doctrinal teachings, Hallisey joins the Sinhalese novelist Wickramasinghe and others who call for attention to the *poetry* of this collection as a guide to their powerful message. In this way, the meaning I am drawing here is less from a literal rendering but from that which appears "between the lines."

36. Here I want to bring attention particularly to what Foucault describes as beginning in the fourth and fifth centuries in Christian spiritual and monastic practice. Foucault also traces self-contemplation forms from Greco-Roman philosophy; his use of "conscience" in these sources is, while relevant, beyond the scope of the current discussion. See Marietta 1970 for a hint at the debate surrounding the existence of an innate faculty of conscience in Stoic philosophy. In relation to the transience of consciousness in Theravada thought, it is compelling that Foucault notes, "In Cassian, perpetual mobility of spirit is the spirit's

weakness. It distracts one from contemplation of God (*First Conference of Abbot Nesterus* 13)"; therefore, "The scrutiny of conscience consists of trying to immobilize consciousness, to eliminate movements of the spirit that divert one from God" (Foucault 1988, 46). It is intriguing to consider how the divine-given capacity for moral discernment in the faculty of the conscience, has become so salient and so implicit in modern theories of mind so as to make other philosophies nearly inconceivable without such a faculty, divinely inspired or not.

37. I do not mean to suggest a static Theravada tradition, nor a unified one. See McDaniel 2008 for a productive and provocative account of pedagogy and change in the Northern Thai tradition. This is also not to suggest that Foucault was wrong in his assessments; he was examining a different tradition. Of course, some argue that Foucault did not go far enough in considering actual bodies; this book as a whole is attempting to mark the social training of bodies, the perceptual coordinates of trained awareness and the lived experience that results in such a dynamic interplay.

3. THE SUBJECTS OF CARE

1. Such ornate accoutrements are admittedly the flourishes of "high-end" conferences. Nevertheless, even rural community meetings will have parallel VIP structures; that is, leaders will be placed at a separate table, and, even in a fan-cooled community hall, the senior (whether by age or other distinction) people in the room will be provided for with distinction.

2. See, for examples, Jackson 2004; Suntaree Komin 1990; Morris 2000; Mulder 2000; Persons 2008a, 2008b; Phillips 1965; Van Esterik 2000.

3. In this discussion, one might find resonance with Eduardo Kohn's notion of the distributed self and "soul blindness," the latter a failure to recognize selves as a cosmic problem in an ecology of selves beyond the human (Kohn 2013). Here, however, I have the more limited concern of elements of the social world training recognition of human attributes.

4. "Group harmony" here refers to the value emergent, and promoted, in these Thai contexts—not a reference to a Durkheimian vision of harmonious societies. A tension should be palpable throughout this chapter, as "harmony" is policed as much as it is spontaneously practiced in this generalized Thai context.

5. In comparing Thai social relations to a body, I risk invoking a conception of bounded collectives, internally changing but nevertheless discrete; it perhaps then must be continually reasserted that these relations can best be understood as transient groupings, with ever-changing margins at all orders of magnitude.

6. These are not perfect divisions; overlap certainly can be found. For work along the Husserl-Merleau-Ponty-Bourdieu trajectory, see, for example, Csordas 1993; see also Throop and Murphy 2002. Zigon 2009b and Mattingly 1998 are prime examples of a Heideggerian take; see Desjarlais 1997 and Good 1994 and 2010 for more Schutz and Foucault influence (among others) within a contemporary phenomenological frame.

7. I am grateful to Wirun Limsawart for drawing my attention to *khwan* in this regard. Shigeharu Tanabe describes the *khwan* as the "soul entity." Further, "The firm unity of the soul entity and body provides health, while the drifting away of soul from body that could occur upon intrusion of external power, or through interference from other influential forces, can result in ill-health or even death" (Tanabe 1991, 186). In defining *khwan* as "soul" or "spirit," Tanabe may evoke a Cartesian duality or even a Christian sensibility inappropriate for this Thai concept. Erik Davis (2016) brings attention to a parallel understanding in Cambodia in a less fraught manner. The 1982 Royal Thai Institute dictionary likens the *khwan* to the spirit, with examples that it can be frightened out of one's body, and it is in this manner that I use the term.

8. Buddhist kings of Southeast Asia traditionally took up the central place in the symbolic architecture of the cosmos and served as ruler by what Heine-Geldern called "the magic of parallelism" (1956, 10). That is, the king rules the state just as the cosmos is ruled by its central source; in turn, the spirit of the collective body is embodied in a leader just as one's individual body is governed by one's spirit or *khwan*.

9. Leadership of the collective parallels the "I" of an individual, though I conceive of bodies on all levels as "selfless selves." That is, no central processing unit is necessary, though well-worn paths constructed through experience develop into perceptions of naturalized units of control.

10. It is difficult for me to imagine what this understanding of reality is like, and an attempt to make these points may conjure romantic or colonialist renderings of "the other." Nevertheless, it could be argued that these spiritual understandings are some of the most intimate aspects of life, as they guide people's actions. Of course, these days many of these ideas (*khwan*, *chata*, and the like) are often rendered as superstition, and many people struggle against such outdated modes of understanding as they seek to embrace scientific renderings of the world. Thus, divulging spiritual convictions, in the way described, risks not only placing oneself in a "lesser" position in what Herzfeld (2003) has called the "global hierarchy of value," but also baring one's level of religious attainment for all to judge. I say this is intimate because of how people shared about such topics with me. Several times, people confided in me "things they had never shared with anyone." But this did not arise with, for instance, the sharing of feelings or displays of grief. Rather, it occurred most frequently when describing something seen during a meditation or times when Buddhist icons had spoken to them. To be frank, this is tentative ground; I do not mean to put my interlocutors in another tense (a la Fabian 1983 and, more recently, Povinelli 2011)—though I am trying to tease out conceptions that flavor things, even when "modern" people actively strive against them.

11. Despite possible drawbacks, I use equilibrium, harmony, and cohesion as synonyms.

12. Varela, Rosch, and Thomspon (1992) draw on Buddhist notions of nondualism from the Madhyamika philosophy of Nagarjuna and mindfulness meditation to reorient cognitive science through a theory of cognition as embodied action. Descola writes of this work in *Beyond Nature and Culture* (2013), calling it "one of the most novel attempts to bypass [the] standoff between a computational interior and an already-structured exterior" characteristic of "Naturalism's" modern mind-body dualism (185). Interesting to note that Descola highlights their use of gestalt psychology but not their use of continental phenomenologists or their explicit use (outside of so-called naturalism's bounds) of Buddhist philosophy. This is particularly striking as Varela, Rosch, and Thompson claim that "the rediscovery of Asian philosophy, particularly of the Buddhist tradition, is a second renaissance in the cultural history of the West, with the potential to be equally important as the rediscovery of Greek thought in the European renaissance" (1992, 22).

13. That is why we also have to understand the nature of the "self" or even the "body" to which we casually refer. As demonstrated, there is a parallel logic to be found between the processing of perceptions at a basic level and the interactions of individuals together in social space. With no homunculus directing the moves, no conscience on which to rely for a sense of moral agency (see chapter 2), ethical action emerges in and from habituation.

14. Raising a *wai* to one's forehead is generally reserved for sacred beings or objects, in which the *wai* is certainly not returned.

15. See Goffman 1955; Hu 1944; Ting-Toomey 1994.

16. *Bun khun* bears some similarity to *guanxi* in this regard, though the differences are beyond the scope of this work.

17. Kleinman and Kleinman make a similar move with a triad of concepts. As they write, "Families, face and favor, then, are not simply social categories, but denote social, psychological and sociosomatic *processes* that enfold moral meaning into persons and that reciprocally project persons into social space" (1993, 39, emphasis original).

18. Sanit Samarkangaan 1975 (สนิท สมัครการ).

19. See Flanders 2011; Suntaree Komin 1990; Persons 2008a, 2008b; Ukosakul 2003.

20. Sanit's article was written in the 1970s, and thus the particular means for face promotion may very well have changed since that time. (Indeed, the Thai physicians described above may serve as a clear illustration of Sanit's logic precisely because they have been away from the country for so long.) Sanit himself argues for a reconsideration of face-making, and his recommendations mirror that of contemporary Buddhist-based social-change advocates, including Phra Paisal's Phuthikā Network.

21. Indeed, Thais are generally considered the quintessential diplomats, and Thailand recently ranked second in the world for service (behind Japan), according to Nate Silver (2011).

22. "คนยากจนก็ไม่ใช่คน "มีหน้ามีตา" เท่าไรอยู่แล้ว เมื่อไม่ใครมีหน้ามีตาการกระทำต่างๆ เพื่อ "รักษาหน้า" ก็ย่อม จะน้อยกว่าเป็นธรรมดา." The particular phrase to represent "face" here (*mī nā mī tā*) can also be parsed as one who is "reputable." Other scholars interested in Thai face, chief among them Larry Persons, have also found wealth to be a strong indicator of face and, by extension, a marker of virtue (see Persons 2008a, 2008b). Persons' work explores the function of face among Thai leadership, and thus he does not delve into whether or not poor people can trade in this form of social capital.

23. Although Flanders (2011) references Sanit in his book, he makes no mention of the parallel here. He draws from Sanit only the correlation between "face" and ego or personality.

24. It may be noteworthy that Flanders (2011) interviewed affluent Bangkokians for his study; so while thirty-nine people eventually admitted that everyone possessed face (fifteen maintaining that only some did), the "everyone" could be a peer set, so the issue remains unclear.

25. William Goode has marked the tendency toward egalitarian ideals in modern scholarship, due to sentimentality and "false nostalgia" (Goode 1978, 356). See also Fischer 2012 for an extended discussion of egalitarianism in scholarship.

26. Investigating in this manner does not mean assuredness that these coordinates will not change; but a would-be radicalism is as romantic as conservatism if it cannot acknowledge the operations of power.

27. I thank Bob Bickner, professor of Thai language and literature at the University of Wisconsin–Madison, for alerting me to this telling phrase (personal correspondence, July 2011). Future research might ascertain when "harmony" entered into Thai political discourse, as does Puett's in the Chinese context (Puett 2012).

28. The Thai word for leader is *hūa nā* (หัวหน้า), literally a combination of head and face.

29. William Goode defines prestige as *"the esteem, respect, or approval that is granted by an individual or collectivity for performances or qualities they consider above the average"* (Goode 1978, 7, emphasis original).

30. William Goode traces the "principles of distributive justice" to the ideas of Aristotle in ancient Greek philosophy through notions of "equity" in the world of social psychology. The Gautama Buddha predates Aristotle by a couple of hundred years, though perhaps it is worth noting the more or less concurrent origins of two different philosophical traditions, the Buddhist tradition being arguably more relevant to the social world of Southeast Asia.

31. Graeber takes up the issue of manners—particularly the opposing interaction styles of avoidance and joking—in order to understand "how forms of social domination come to be experienced in the most intimate possible ways" (Graeber 2007, 16). Graeber is also explor-

ing the roots of capitalism and market exchange in relation to these interaction styles. The principle of avoidance is here based on the idea that certain groups or individuals are sacred, while the principle of joking is based on bodies being one common substance. At the risk of defiling the basis of his argument, I will leave off these aspects of his discussion at this time.

32. Indeed, the metaphor only goes so far. Certainly the gall bladder does not complain behind the heart's back, drag its feet on the way to meetings, manipulate the heart by giving partial or false reports, or fail to cooperate at all. My thanks to Eli Elinoff for making this point with such humor.

33. As Graeber puts it, "How often, for instance, does one hear the upper classes of some society or other described as more refined and elegant than those below them, finer in features, more tactful and disciplined in their emotions? Or hear that the lower orders are cruder, coarser in features as in manners—but at the same time more free with their feelings, more spontaneous? Most people seem to consider it a matter of course that upper and lower stratum of society should differ in this way (if they think about it at all, perhaps they write it off to conditions of health, work, and leisure), or at least, that they should be represented so" (Graeber 2007, 27). Certainly anyone familiar with Thailand will hear a familiar division, whether expressed between the urban and the rural, the city and the countryside, the rich and the poor. Even the color of one's skin bears the marks of society's presumptions—and the number of skin-whitening products attests to the understanding that a change in the surface can actually serve to change others' presumptions and, in turn, one's social position.

34. See Fassin 2008; Laidlaw 2002; Zigon 2008.

35. Interesting to note, Sanit (สนิท สมัครการ 1975) provides examples for face-promoting activities, including volunteering (kan`āsā or rap`āsā) alongside arranging ceremonies and giving money to the poor. Sanit even names volunteering as a means to increase, and of course evidence of, "face" at the national level as well, suggesting that a high rate of volunteerism, like hosting international meetings, is an important indicator of prestige of the nation.

36. Heim in turn calls for moral anthropology to pay close attention to the way people perceive, as noted above.

4. THE CIVIC LANDSCAPE OF CARE

1. See ลือชัย ศรีเงินยวง และ ยงยุทธ พงษ์สุภาพ 2009.

2. "Laws Concerning Volunteers and Giving" (กฎหมายที่เกี่ยวข้องกับอาสาสมัครและการให้, published by สถาบันไทยรูรัลเน็ต, Thai Rural Net 2550 (2007) attempts to review the historical trends in volunteering and the policies that have helped define its practice. This publication, part of the library of the Volunteer Spirit Network, is indicative of renewed interest in volunteerism and attempts to reinvigorate the prominence and moral valence of organized social action.

3. One of the biggest models for Thai volunteers at the turn of the century was the Red Cross. The Siamese Red Cross Society was established in 1893, under patronage of the king. After the abolition of the absolute monarchy in 1932, Thailand's volunteer organizations were few, though a handful of important groups arose in those days, with emphasis placed on bringing help to the countryside from urban centers (e.g., Dr. Puey Ungphakorn's Thammasat Graduate Volunteers). The 1973 student-led revolution for democracy seemed to usher in an increase in volunteer activity, only to be drastically lessened following the military crackdown of 1976. Nevertheless, through the 1980s, volunteer groups increased. Of particular note, the Thai Volunteer Service formed in 1980 with the explicit purpose of raising the consciousness of young people and developing Thai society.

4. The Thai Rural Net's treatise is not an attempt to trace the rise of čhit`āsā; on the contrary, it seems largely geared to promoting such a change in emphasis. Perhaps future

archival work could help pinpoint the increased prominence of the word *čhit`āsā*. I cannot be certain it does not appear in volunteer platforms prior to 2001—though it certainly does not appear in any of the laws and policies outlined by the Thai Rural Net before 2004. People seem to agree this is a new term, and I have heard tell that it is finding its way into many factions of Thai society, from the type of government workers described here to motorcycle taxi associations (Sopranzetti, personal communication). In the discussion of the Volunteer Spirit Network in this chapter, I trace one possible source of the term, as propagated by a key leader in this network.

5. There are sometimes caveats to these basic determinants, such as those that demand volunteers are gainfully employed elsewhere (in the context of volunteer probation, out of the Ministry of Justice, บริบทของอาสาสมัครคุมประพฤติ กระทรวงยุติธรรม), or those that clarify volunteers can be within both government and public welfare organizations (as according to the 2003 Royal Act to Support the Welfare of Society, พระราชบัญญัติ ส่งเสริมการจัดสวัสดิการสังคม).

6. See Putnam 2000. The TRN may be understood to agree with this sentiment. But the association between volunteerism and democracy is not without contention, and debates about voluntary civic engagement rage in political science; for an account that places volunteerism at the heart of American democratic organizing, see Stout's 2010 *Blessed Are the Organized*.

7. The Department of Social Welfare: *krom prachāsongkhrǫ*, กรมประชาสงเคราะห์). See คณะ รัฐมนตรีชุดพลเอก สุรยุทธ์ จุลานนท์ 2007 for details of initial assessment. According to research conducted in 2006, about 459,140 older people live alone—approximately 7.1 percent of the population over the age of sixty-five.

8. The pilot program included eight provinces: Petchaburi and Supanaburi (Central region), Konkaen and Roiet (Northeast), Chiangmai and Pitsanulok (North), and Sonklaa and Suraattaani (South).

9. My translation; see คณะรัฐมนตรีชุดพลเอก สุรยุทธ์ จุลานนท์ 2007.

10. See details: http://www.chainat.m-society.go.th/volun-agde.htm (pdf available).

11. See Ellis and Noyes 1978. Even hospice volunteers—who are mandated to conduct 5 percent of hospice work in the United States—are restricted in their care provision by strict laws governing what tasks volunteers can perform. Litigation concerns fuel these restrictions; as a telling example, hospice volunteers are not permitted to lift a patient who has fallen in the home during their visit.

12. Bree's work began in 2005, under the auspices of the Project to Prepare for an Aging Society of the MSDHS: *khrōngkān trīam khwāmphrǭm sū sangkhom phūsūng`āiyu* (โครงการเตรียมความพร้อมสู่สังคมผู้สูงอายุ). The volunteer program is in fact one of six parts of this project, which also includes preparing those aged forty-five to sixty for old age, working with families of older people, renovating houses for poor older people, creating community savings initiatives, and harnessing the wisdom of older people for social good.

13. It is likely that the public health Aw Saw Maw volunteers began in exactly the same fashion—a network of people able to distribute important information, tools, and skills to their families through connection with the public health ministry. The future remains uncertain, then, for the volunteers for the elderly, for whom success could spell increasing governmental demands.

14. This echoes common conceptions of ideal village life, in which solidarity and reciprocity are at the heart of a local sufficiency economy, complete with a humanitarian—rather than capitalist—base (Chaitthip Nartsupha 1991; Baker and Pasuk 1999; Reynolds 2009). For further critique of this mystique, see Kemp 1988 and Vandergeest 1996. For a more generalized critique of egalitarian projections, see Fischer 2012.

15. OPO's work at the time of my research also included income-generating projects, social welfare advocacy, and the support of elder person clubs. The mission of OPO is strongly influenced by the agenda of HelpAge International, and because of the Thai

government's top-down instillation of many programs that map onto HelpAge goals (including, for instance, the establishment of elder person clubs in every district of every county), Thailand is in many ways a poster child (and inspiration) for HelpAge's work. OPO sees its work as making the international goals "culturally appropriate," and in empowering people to have greater investment in what otherwise could be merely bureaucratically organized government programs.

16. There was only one volunteer who visited Aom and her family nearly every day of their mother's protracted illness. Amaa was an eighty-five-year-old woman (they do not actually know her real name, calling her instead by the Northern Thai term for grandma), and she came each day for approximately thirty minutes to perform "Yoray" energy healing on Tatsanii and Ying. Yoray attracts practitioners with claims of unlocking people's power to heal by using their hands. Although Yoray is a fairly recent phenomenon in Thailand (with allegedly Japanese roots), it nonetheless entails a set task that provides Amaa a somewhat understandable and specific entrée into the household. It is a modeled physical behavior, including the raising of a hand as a conduit for healing energy. And while accompanied by scandalous accusations of being a pyramid scheme (Yoray practitioners are pressured to make donations, buy pendants, recruit family members, and ultimately dissociate with those who refuse to join), it nevertheless provides something lacking in other schemes.

17. Wealthier people do not readily fit into volunteer schemas. On the way back to the Chiang Mai city center on our Aw Paw Saw foray, for instance, Bree and our company drove by a walled and gated suburban housing complex, rising up out of the landscape with paddy fields on one side and the edges of an industrial satellite city on the other. It certainly stood in stark contrast to typical village life, with so much enclosure, house after house. And indeed, the government does not try to penetrate those spaces: it is too difficult to get volunteers in, they say. But the class divide evident here is a common theme in volunteer programs. Like the Aw Saw Maw public health volunteers before them, the Aw Paw Saw draw mainly from the lower classes: crudely put, poor people taking care of poorer people. Social scientists have commented on the need to bridge the class divide in volunteerism in the future (see โกมาตร จึงเสถียรทรัพย์ [Komatra Cheungsatiansup] et al. 2550 [2007]), but rarely from the close vantage point of the operations of pity. At least it is fair to say that the organizers of government volunteers for older people are unconcerned with people in gated communities, and it is hard to find a group of volunteers interested in helping the rich and resourced.

18. I certainly talked with men who were caring for their parents; these men often mentioned such stereotypes, and they seemed to take pride in their abilities to provide care, despite their gender "handicap."

19. This could alternately be translated as the Spirit of Volunteering Network; I opt here for the more concise title, at the risk of obscuring the spirit of the term. There are influences to the spirit of volunteering movement other than those I emphasize here, including the Taiwanese Buddhist Tsu Chi model. For Buddhist lineages associated with the movement, as well as a repetition of the common genesis story, see สุธาทิพย์ แก้วเกลี้ยง 2006. For promotional stories of the spirit of volunteering, see จารุประภา วะสี และ มัณฑนา บรรณาธรรม nd.

20. This was not an entirely new idea. Research conducted well before the tsunami, including Juree Vichit-Vadakan's 2002 piece titled *An Overview of Philanthropy and Civil Society in Thailand* (found in the Volunteer Spirit Network library) indicates an attempt by research bodies in Thailand to understand typical Thai patterns of philanthropy—particularly the tendency for donations to Buddhist temples—in order to promote more grassroots funding of civil society organizations.

21. See www.volunteerspirit.org.

22. Future research is needed to pinpoint the term's derivation and utilization.

23. P. A. Payutto 2001 and Buddhadasa 1992 are prime examples; see also Streckfuss 2011, 249.

24. In Simpkins' powerful analysis (2003), she calls this move a "draw"—although it demanded NGOs communicate with the government and thus increased the central government's knowledge of local activities, it also granted increased legitimacy for smaller NGOs.

25. On the invention of tradition, see Reynolds 2009, Streckfuss 2011, Thongchai 1994, and Hamilton 1991. Of note: the twelfth of these decrees involved protecting children, the elderly, and the handicapped.

26. Wichit Wichitwathakan (วิจิตรวิจิตรวาทการ), also known as Luang Wichitwathakan.

27. This influx of new Thai words occurred at the same time as the country known as Siam was renamed Thailand. It was a time of heavy "culture mandates," and as Streckfuss contends, "Many of today's Thai believe that the 'invented traditions' of this period are authentic Thai customs" (Streckfuss 2011, 233). This is also linked to a major issue for Thai studies, namely the vague quality known as *khwām pen thai* (ความเป็นไทย), or Thai-ness, that, although best described in terms of what it is not, rather than what it is, is claimed to be an essence incomprehensible to foreigners (see Thongchai 1994, 7–8).

28. Instead, according to Amara Pongsapich, the Thai National Human Rights commissioner, small groups came together under the radar of the central government to demand "radical reforms to stop the alleged transfer of national resources from the poorer to the wealthier sectors of Thai society" (Yamamoto 1995, 246).

29. Acceptability standards, not to mention the somewhat mandatory expense of police bribes to speed the registration process and so forth (see Simpkins 2003, 266).

30. The boards of some NGOs function mainly as a formality, providing very little in the way of organizational direction or evaluation. In one board meeting I attended, the agenda was set to review the organization's strategic plan; board members took turns identifying spelling errors in the circulated document or talking at length about their own (unrelated) works in local communities.

31. Simpkins, in her incisive analysis of NGO activity, recounts, "In the mid 1980s, there were less than twenty major Thai NGOs. These included the Thai Rural Reconstruction Movement, Thai Volunteer Service, Catholic credit union groups, and some slum organizations such as the renowned Duang Prateep in Bangkok" (Simpkins 2003, 282–283).

32. Simpkins too notes this categorization from Hirsch's 1991 *Development Dilemmas in Rural Thailand* (see Simpkins 2003, 259).

33. See Simpkins (2003, 257 and 271) for more details.

34. As it was explained to me by governmental and nongovernmental personnel alike, there are roughly two career paths for social work graduates: students enter either the government track for positions in the Ministry of Social Development or related departments, or they aim to enter the NGO track. The TVS places people interested in the latter for two-year internship-type positions—with approximately 40–50 percent of these trainees remaining with NGOs on a long-term basis, many in leadership positions. (See www .gnh-movement.org/followup_detail.php?id=139 for more information.)

TVS promotional materials claim key activist gains for former TVS volunteers in all regions of the country except the South. There is much to speculate about such an important exception. As the director of OPO explained to me, Southern workers are "very strong" and refuse to bend to government pressure, and in turn, fail to play by the unofficial rules of the NGO game. He went on to give an example of a women's group who created a very successful income-generating project bottling a special chili sauce. A government official from the agriculture department came to inspect their operations and claimed they needed to have official recognition, ensuring the public that their product was not dangerous— that is, he demanded 4,000 baht payment for a sticker pronouncing their chili a "Product of the Agricultural Department." The leader of the women's collective vehemently refused ("a sticker for what?!"), causing a rift between the organization and the government, eventually leading to the destruction of the project. This example highlights the way government ministries attempt to put their stamps on successful community projects, claiming some modicum of success for themselves, as well as the need for these small organizations to have powerful advocates in their ranks to protect their efforts and lend legitimacy to their organizations. The predominantly Muslim southern region has a long history of struggles for independence from the predominantly Buddhist power centers of Thailand, and the refusal to join in the patronage system here reflects the power and perils of such a choice.

35. Again, stigma results from assessments of NGOs as both overly conservative and overly radical elements in Thai society. NGO numbers seem to rise and fall with economic ebbs and flows. When the economy is booming, many people join the more lucrative private sector; when crises hit, larger numbers are attracted to grassroots efforts. However you slice it, this is a relatively small world. The TVS claims that, since 1980, they have recruited and trained only five hundred full-time volunteers; nevertheless, given the high stakes of such involvement, this somewhat marginal group seems to have made a large impression on Thai popular opinion.

36. OPO, in its role implementing the volunteers for the elder program, borders on a GONGO in this regard. The stigma of profiteering government volunteering remains, but in a less politically contentious manner.

37. คำ ผกา "ไม่เถียงแต่ด่า" มติชน สุดสัปดาห์ (3–9 ก.ย.53). Kam Pagaa's article is not the first in this series. It began with a criticism of Phra Paisal from the writer Pakavadee (no surname), whose comments can be seen as the antecedents to Kam Pagaa's argument: see http://www.prachatai.com/journal/2010/08/30801 for her article, "Phra Paisal Wisalo: Reform Autocracy—'Abhisit' Must Dare to Lead Change" (พระไพศาล วิสาโล: ปฏิรูปอัตตาธิปไตย —'อภิสิทธิ์ ต้องกล้านำความเปลียนแปลง). Phra Paisal responded in an open letter to Khun Pakavadee (http://www.visalo.org/article/letterToPakawadee.htm, last accessed December 2018), launching the series of articles to which I refer here.

38. Kam Pagaa defends herself in this regard by arguing that monks should not be above criticism; she claims that to hold monks in such high regard as to keep them above critique is a modern middle-class phenomenon, and that, in the countryside at least, people discuss and condemn the actions of monks freely.

39. Krathoo Dokthong, or "slut agenda," comes from the Lanna language slang term *dokthong*, literally "golden flower."

40. The details of this controversial political situation are beyond the scope of this chapter. Refer to the introduction for background; more discussion on the political fault lines appear in chapter 5.

41. For this quotation, Kam Pagaa refers to an open letter Phra Paisal published in the journal *K Kon* and on his website; see http://www.visalo.org/article/letterToPakawadee .htm.

42. In Thai: *næo rūam prachāthiptai tǭtān phadetkānhængchāt*, แนวร่วมประชาธิปไตยต่อ ด้านเผด็จการแห่งชาติ or นปช.

43. Interestingly, Phra Paisal was not quoting a Buddhist source but rather Adam Kahane, author of *Power and Love: A Theory and Practice of Social Change*.

44. Phra Paisal also discusses structure in other ways: not so much in terms of the structural violence Kam Pagaa addresses in terms of systematic oppression and disenfranchisement by the elite and ordained upper echelons of society, but in terms of the structural changes occurring in Thailand that have ushered in greater political participation of the lower classes. He thus contends that poor and lower-middle-class Thai people are no longer willing to put up with disparity as they did in the past. It should be noted further that while Kam Pagaa, a feminist Marxist thinker, does well to call out the power structure

associated with dharmic "truth-beyond-truth," ironically she too draws on the presumption of special knowledge. She intimates that she and her fellow intellectuals can see clearly while others are left either with conniving power trips or false consciousness. Phra Paisal may in contrast be seen to admit more nuance, or at least retain more flexibility, through his partial acknowledgement of the issue of structural violence.

45. Streckfuss is greatly indebted to Christine Gray's pioneering work on the generation of "a new Buddhist aristocracy" disguised in a variety of ways but depending on expanding royal merit.

5. THE VIOLENCE OF CARE

1. *Real Life Dramas 84000* or *lakhǫn chīwit čhing chut 84000* (ละครชีวิตจริงชุด 84000). The numerical title has religious significance: as the Buddha, often referred to as the Great Physician, "prescribed 84,000 antidotes for the 84,000 afflictions of living beings." All aim toward ending ignorance (see http://online.sfsu.edu/~rone/Buddhism/Inner%20Ecology.htm).

2. Charles Keyes once noted, "In popular Buddhism, that is, among practicing Theravada Buddhists, karma is invoked as an explanation of conditions that have emerged in one's lifetime only on rare occasions" (1983, 265). It was my experience too that oftentimes people would assume untraceable past lives were at the heart of their current experience (for better or worse), though this program clearly presents what may in fact be a growing focus on "fast karma." However, even more important may be the *process* of training awareness on karmic explanations.

3. Boonyuang had once laughingly characterized visitors by ethnicity to me—the Chinese, she had said, come over for three minutes and then go, in contrast to the leisurely chatting and just being of the Northern Thai, and I could only assume at that point that a foreigner like me was more akin in her mind to the Chinese.

4. This clearly suggests there are positive psychological effects at play even amid overt justification for and erasure of oppression. But the implications of "alternative models for personal agency" that Cassaniti (2015) claims have yet to be fully mapped. This is meant to begin such a discussion.

5. See Jackson 1989 and 2016; Sinnott 2004. There is a violent underside to what is otherwise known as Asia's "Gay Capital." Discrimination is on the rise, documented by academics, journalists, and activists alike (see https://asiancorrespondent.com/2014/03/rising-lgbt-discrimination-challenges-thailands-culture-of-tolerance/, last accessed March 30, 2018). There were troubling signs that the Red Shirts in the North were casting trans* communities as "other," to be cast out of their ideal movement; the Chiang Mai 51, for instance, was accused of gay-bashing at a political protest rally the same month this episode aired.

6. This was at least true during the time of my primary research; ten years later, Pailin is suffering from the turn to digital outlets, as one retailer told me, and their bookracks are far less prevalent.

7. An alternative translation is "Damn Revenge" (by Nop Nanthawan, นพ นันทวัน). The title also conjures *čhaokamnāiwēn*, the actual incarnation of a karmic presence, a person or a ghost, that plagues you.

8. Abortion is legal in Thailand only in instances of rape and when the mother's life is endangered. The reasons for abortion are left out of the clear stance on the issue taken in the book.

9. DNA กรรม, ราช รามัญ 2008.

10. Like Bowie (1998), demonstrating the manipulation of the rich by the poor through merit-making, Jordt shows "the very significant role monks and laity play in shaping the terms of political legitimation through apolitical actions" (Jordt 2007, 13).

11. Indeed, the founding of Bangkok included a massive attempt by the elite to expunge the supernatural elements of Buddhist practice without ever achieving a clear resolution (see Baker and Pasuk Phongpaichit 2017, particularly pages 202 and 274). One might see resonance with what Herzfeld (2002) calls "crypto-colonialism" in this regard, insofar as the elite aimed to capture the far reaches of the recongealing kingdom with a uniform national culture, but the terms of the debate are by no means completely the result of Western models and dependencies.

12. This is not to suggest that what I characterize as a "cosmopolitan" or "progressive" view is either more recent or less authentic.

13. "นิสัยคนไทยเป็นคนเอื้อเฟื้อเผื่อแผ่ คนไทยจะไม่ชอบให้ใครบังคับ"

14. As Brapin expressed it, "60 percent ที่มาด้วยใจแล้วก็ทำงานด้วยความตั้งใจ"

15. To be clear, I am not intimating that this is the truth per se, but this instance speaks to widespread presumptions and part of what we might call, following Julie Livingston and others, the "collective moral imaginary" (Livingston 2012), the roots of which I am attempting to unearth.

16. *Mettā* is one of the four sublime states (*brahmavihāras*) described in Theravada Buddhist scriptures, most commonly translated as "loving-kindness." Other translations include friendliness, benevolence, kindness, love, sympathy, and active interest in others. (Previously in the text, *kwammettā* was used, the noun form related to this Buddhist value/ principle.) *Mettā* (เมตตา) is the first of four sublime states, along with *karunā* (กรุณา, compassion or mercy), *muthitā* (มุทิตา, sympathetic joy), and `*ubēkkhā* (อุเบกขา, equanimity). Also underlying this pity is a broadly understood notion of karma—general laws of cause and effect that span lifetimes: so you might pity someone's karmic baggage, so to speak; or the poor wise man can pity the rich fool.

17. This was not a hidden sentiment. The interview from which I draw Brapin's quotes was conducted in the open area of a home for the disabled, surrounded by people in wheelchairs and other forms of dependency that elicit similar "pity."

18. While I am not claiming a systematic linguistic analysis here, I might also note "love," too, could use some unpacking, analytically and phenomenologically. Take, for instance, the "love" referred to by radical social movements (with reference to the Reverend Dr. Martin Luther King Jr. and Che Guevara, among others): To what state do these calls refer, and how is one trained to perceive the world in this way? Maria Heim (2017, Oxford Handbook of Indian Philosophy) offers a reading on Buddhaghosa's phenomenology of love and compassion of note in this regard.

19. Thus the "Four Noble Truths": suffering, the cause of suffering, the cessation of suffering, and the eight-fold path.

20. The term "idiot compassion" would thus refer to moves to "help" others without a basic understanding of the root cause of suffering, resulting in the furthering of worldly attachments and a placating or worsening of suffering. One might consult Hallisey and Saddhatissa's introductory *Buddhist Ethics* (1997) as a guide to overarching ethical frames, though I generally find reference to "Buddhism" as such unhelpful.

21. Stein was Husserl's student, though her work, while no less groundbreaking, has been less celebrated than some of his other students. Some have wondered what course phenomenology, and European academe in general, would have taken had Stein, a woman and a Jew, been his heir-apparent rather than Heidegger. See Sawicki 1998 for a great introduction/interpretation of her work and its importance.

22. Although some recent work on empathy utilizes parts of Stein, this basic element is less emphasized than her ideas regarding embodiment. See Throop 2008.

23. One might wonder what Edith Stein would have gotten from the Abhidhamma in this regard, as its theory of mind sets up the coordinates of such interpersonal influence. Indeed, as Sawicki (1998) assesses, Stein took to the Catholic nunnery after she failed to

secure a post in the European academy to explore exactly how external influence—which she took to by necessity be divine—could be ascertained and studied further.

24. If pity holds inflections of inferiority in one way or another—whether cast simply as bad luck or more as inborn traits—it may be fine to articulate in some ethical frames but is anathema to egalitarian ethics. In this way, this analysis is not limited to the Thai context. Despite certain ambivalences, international humanitarian logic—as Miriam Ticktin, Didier Fassin, and others have explored—requires a victim status for beneficiaries of humanitarianism, which one could argue maps onto pity as well. And this has arisen despite historical rhetoric of solidarity and egalitarianism. The imperialist roots of the Western world in full ironic bloom?

25. Some saw the introduction of a Patient's Bill of Rights as a first step toward a litigious medical system, opening the door to conceptions of (and lawsuits claiming) medical malpractice. For discussion of the Patient's Bill of Rights, its ethical ramifications, and interpersonal effects, see Stonington 2009.

26. Reeler (1996), for example, offers possible modes of empowerment in changing health-care relationships; Wheeler (2010) provides a more cynical perspective.

27. This seems to have particularly been the case in the early years of the program, when such a connection provided people with special health-care access and the program was a vital link to health information and other resources. In general, Somkiati claimed others would still find such a connection a reliable source of status, though when pressed, he admitted the opposite could be the case (if, for instance, a volunteer was perceived as fame-mongering or ladder-climbing).

28. *Khrūa* (เครือ) has a variety of definitions, including a vine or creeping plant, and a bunch of bananas.

29. In this regard, there are similarities between this group and the community of Pom Mahakan in Bangkok, the subject of Michael Herzfeld's work in Thailand for many years (Herzfeld 2016).

30. NGOs are often presumed allies of the poor and underserved in global public health rhetoric; however, it is also often true that global public health promoters collaborate with autocratic regimes and engaged undemocratic processes in the quest for health equity.

31. The UDD Red Shirts had one central demand from 2008 to 2011: the dissolution of parliament and the holding of new elections. Opposition to such a vote was fueled by a distrust of popular sentiment. In an article published on the heels of the violent government crackdown on protesters in Bangkok May 2011, the geographer Jim Glassman captured such a sentiment in a quote from a PAD supporter who participated in the 2008 airport takeover: "Rural people have good hearts but they don't know the truth like we do in Bangkok. It is our duty to re-educate them" (Glassman 2011, 43; for quote in original context, see Bloomberg.com, December 1, 2008). But it must be noted that political conservatism is not synonymous with neoliberal economic reform efforts, as is often the case elsewhere. There is a strange mixing of bedfellows in the political factions in Thailand today, as discussed in the introduction, with "revolutionary" figures of the Red Shirts seeing freedom and progress in consumer-based systems of development, while political conservatives echo global activist rally cries against capitalism and its motives.

32. Rural etiquette might be a factor here as well. Northern "country" people do not stand on airs in the same way that urban and central Thais generally do, and there may be a mixing of patterns occurring with these political affiliations. It is also important to note that although protests provide a forum for complaint, both Yellow and Red gatherings were remarkable for their overall peaceful and jovial feel—with music, markets, and meals shared in good spirits. For analysis of the narrative forms animating the scene in the bakeshop, as well as care given and received amid precarity, see Aulino forthcoming.

33. August 23, 2011, http://enews.mcot.net/view.php?id=11460, accessed March 30, 2012.

34. As the article reported, the spokesman for the royalist Democrat Party was clear: "Every political party must help reduce social conflicts because the country will be at a dead-end again 'if politics is played outside Parliament.'"

35. On General Prem's birthday in August 2009, not only did Red Shirt supporters dress in black, I heard tell of full-length funeral proceedings held for him in Chiang Mai, a powerful ritually fueled symbolic gesture, akin perhaps to burning him in effigy.

36. As translated on the Australia National University's Southeast Asia blog *New Mandala*, August 4, 2011, http://asiapacific.anu.edu/newmandala/wp-content/uploads/2011/08/Slogan.jpg. Original Thai available at https://www.newmandala.org/royal-motherhood-statement/slogan/.

37. See Glassman 2011 for a review, cf. McCargo 2005.

38. Taking this allusion to the Lernaean Hydra to the extreme, it might seem that those in the "old guard" who repeatedly condone violence against protesters believe it necessary to cut off all these new heads (that is, all those Red-leaning elected leaders and local would-be leaders) to kill the beast.

39. On August 26, 2009, popular political blog *The BKK Pundit* reported the following: "In the last few days, AC Nielson released a survey/report showing that in July the PM's Office was the third largest advertiser in the media and in total spent 160 million Baht. This is double, the 76 million Baht, spent in June. In just two months, the PM's Office has spent 236 million Baht on advertising." Further, "This is just the advertising from one government agency and doesn't include all the advertising of government departments/ministries and of Bangkok Governor." It also must pale in comparison to resources dedicated to the weekly national addresses given by the acting prime minister general, some of which go on for hours.

CONCLUSION

1. Maria Heim (2014) claims that the Jatakas illustrate and develop Buddhist teachings in important ways. Speaking in a register different from other parts of the Pali Canon, these narratives show how Buddhist philosophy and moral codes of conduct play out in people's lives, however fantastical some of the stories may seem. For more on how people speak and perform according to Theravadin narrative forms, see Aulino forthcoming.

2. McMahan (2008) describes this type of analysis as a modernist interpretation of interdependence found in Thich Nhat Hanh's *The Heart of Understanding: Commentaries on the Prajnaparamita Heart Sutra*. As he surmises, the intention is "to encourage society to take responsibility for the plight of the disadvantaged, not to reformulate the doctrine of karma" (McMahan 2008, 175).

3. These frameworks are incredibly helpful in making visible powerful currents in social worlds, as well as helping manage the complexity of any given situation, but must be used and abandoned and altered as necessary for retaining flexibility and continued creative purpose. Here I resonate with the way Cheryl Mattingly (2014) draws on and yet departs from Aristotle for a first-person virtue ethics, through which she recognizes moral agents as not only responding to but also acting upon history. In framing scenes from everyday life as "moral laboratories" rather than "moral prisons" or illustrations of skeptically derived social theory, she captures a similar sense of "how social change might occur" (203).

4. From Angela Davis's 1989 address at Spelman College, quoted in brown 2017, 4, fn 3.

5. See generativesomatics.org.

6. Puett argues that anthropologists have mistakenly deduced notions of cosmological ontology from ritual, when in fact the theory behind ritual can be geared toward creating

rather than naming. Desjarlais (2016) can be read in a similar way as he traces tantric ritual technologies for the transference of consciousness after death among the Hyolmo in Nepal.

7. Jordt (2007) points to something similar when identifying culturally specific strategies of political legitimization operating in Burma, acknowledging as well how tricky such efforts can be (see chapter 5).

8. For adrienne maree brown, doing can facilitate a learning through experience. This then is part and parcel of "strategies for organizers building movements for justice and liberation that leverage relatively simple interactions to create complex patterns, systems, and transformations—including adaptation, interdependence and decentralization, fractal awareness, resilience and transformative justice, nonlinear and iterative change, creating more possibilities" (brown 2017, 24).

References

Asad, Talal. 1993. *Genealogies of Religion: Discipline and Reasons of Power in Christianity and Islam.* Baltimore: Johns Hopkins University Press.

Ascoli, Ugo, and Costanzo Ranci. 2002. *Dilemmas of the Welfare Mix: The New Structure of Welfare in an Era of Privatization.* New York: Kluwer Academic/Plenum.

Aulino, Felicity. 2014. "Perceiving the Social Body: A Phenomenological Perspective on Ethical Practice in Buddhist Thailand." *Journal of Religious Ethics* 42 (3): 415–441.

Aulino, Felicity. 2017. "Narrating the Future: Population Aging and the Demographic Imaginary in Thailand." *Medical Anthropology* 36 (8).

Aulino, Felicity. Forthcoming. "Everyday Care and Precarity: Buddhaghosa and Thai Social Story-Making." *Medical Anthropology* 39 (2).

Aulino, Felicity, Eli Elinoff, Claudio Sopranzetti, and Benjamin Tausig. 2014. "Fieldsights— Hot Spots: The Wheel of Crisis in Thailand." Cultural Anthropology Online. https://culanth.org/fieldsights/582-the-wheel-of-crisis-in-thailand.

Austin, J. L. 1962. *How to Do Things with Words.* Cambridge, MA: Harvard University Press.

Baker, Chris, and Pasuk Phongpaichit. 1999. *The Thai Village Economy in the Past.* Chiang Mai: Silkworm Press.

Baker, Chris, and Pasuk Phongpaichit. 2017. *A History of Ayutthaya: Siam in the Early Modern World.* Cambridge: Cambridge University Press.

Bayat, Asef. 2013. "The Arab Spring and Its Surprises." *Development and Change* 44 (3): 587–601.

Bell, Catherine. 1992. *Ritual Theory, Ritual Practice.* Oxford: Oxford University Press.

Bell, Catherine. 1997. *Ritual: Perspectives and Dimensions.* New York: Oxford University Press.

Bellah, Robert N. 1994. "Understanding Caring in Contemporary America." In *The Crisis of Care: Affirming and Restoring Caring Practices in the Helping Professions,* edited by S. S. Phillips and P. Benner, 16–30. Washington, DC: Georgetown University Press.

Benner, Patricia E. 1994. "Caring as a Way of Knowing and Not Knowing." In *The Crisis of Care,* edited by S. S. Phillips and P. E. Benner, 42–62. Washington, DC: Georgetown University Press.

Biehl, João. 2012. "Care and Disregard." In *A Companion to Moral Anthropology,* edited by D. Fassin, 242–263. Chichester, UK: Wiley-Blackwell.

Bilmes, Leela. 2001. *Sociolinguistic Aspects of Thai Politeness.* Berkeley: University of California Press.

Blackman, Lisa. 2013. "Habit and Affect: Revitalizing a Forgotten History." *Body and Society* 19 (2/3): 186–216.

Borneman, John. 1997. "Caring and Being Cared For: Displacing Marriage, Kinship, Gender and Sexuality." *International Social Science Journal* 49 (154): 573–584.

Borneman, John, and Abdellah Hammoudi. 2009. *Being There: The Fieldwork Encounter and the Making of Truth.* Berkeley: University of California Press.

Bourdieu, Pierre, and Loic J. D. Wacquant. 1992. *An Invitation to Reflexive Sociology.* Chicago: University of Chicago Press.

Bowie, Katherine. 1998. "The Alchemy of Charity: Of Class and Buddhism in Northern Thailand." *American Anthropologist* 100 (2): 469.

Brahinsky, Josh. 2018. "Effects of Scale: How Western Agency-Anxieties Mold Affect Theory, and How Pentecostalism and Neuroscience Teach Us to Think Differently." *Anthropological Theory* 18 (4): 478–501.

brown, adrienne maree. 2017. *Emergent Strategy: Shaping Change, Changing Worlds*. Chico, CA: AK Press.

Buch, Elana. 2013. "Senses of Care: Embodying Inequality and Sustaining Personhood in the Home Care of Older Adults in Chicago." *American Ethnologist* 40 (4): 637–650.

Buch, Elana. 2015. "Anthropology of Aging and Care." *Annual Review of Anthropology* 44 (1).

Buddhadasa Bhikkhu. 1992. *Paticcasamuppada: Practical Dependent Origination*. Bangkok: Vuddhidhamma Fund.

Burke, Peter. 1987. *The Historical Anthropology of Early Modern Italy: Essays on Perception and Communication*. Cambridge: Cambridge University Press.

Cassaniti, Julia. 2015. *Living Buddhism: Mind, Self, and Emotion in a Thai Community*. Ithaca, NY: Cornell University Press.

Cavell, Stanley. 1986. "The Uncanniness of the Ordinary." In *Tanner Lectures on Human Values*. Stanford, CA: Stanford University Press.

Chaitthip Nartsupha. 1991. "The Community Culture School of Thought." In *Thai Constructions of Knowledge*, edited by Manas Chitakasem and A. Turton, 118–141. London: School of Oriental and African Studies, University of London.

Christakis, Nicholas A. 1999. *Death Foretold: Prophecy and Prognosis in Medical Care*. Chicago: University of Chicago Press.

Ciavolella, Riccardo, and Stefano Boni. 2015. "Aspiring to Alterpolitics: Anthropology, Radical Theory, and Social Movements." *Focaal—Journal of Global and Historical Anthropology* 72:3–8.

Collins, Steven. 2013. *Self and Society: Essays on Pali Literature and Social Theory 1988–2010*. Chiang Mai: Silkworm Books.

Connors, Michael Kelly. 2003. *Democracy and National Identity in Thailand*. New York: RoutledgeCurzon.

Csordas, Thomas. 1993. "Somatic Modes of Attention." *Cultural Anthropology* 8 (2): 135–156.

Danely, Jason. 2015. "Of Technoscapes and Elderscapes: Editor's Commentary on the Special Issue 'Aging the Technoscape.'" *Anthropology and Aging* 36 (2):110–111.

Das, Veena. 2007. *Life and Words: Violence and the Descent into the Ordinary*. Berkeley: University of California Press.

Das, Veena. 2012. "Ordinary Ethics." In *A Companion to Moral Anthropology*, edited by D. Fassin, 133–149. Malden, MA: Wiley Blackwell.

Davis, Erik W. 2016. *Deathpower: Buddhism's Ritual Imagination in Cambodia*. New York: Columbia University Press.

Davis, Richard B. 1984. *Muang Metaphysics: A Study of Northern Thai Myth and Ritual*. Bangkok: Pandora.

Descola, Philippe. 2013. *Beyond Nature and Culture*. Chicago: University of Chicago Press.

Desjarlais, Robert. 1997. *Shelter Blues: Sanity and Selfhood among the Homeless*. Philadelphia: University of Pennsylvania Press.

Desjarlais, Robert. 2003. *Sensory Biographies: Lives and Deaths among Nepal's Yolmo Buddhists*. Berkeley: University of California Press.

Desjarlais, Robert. 2016. *Subject to Death: Life and Loss in a Buddhist World*. Chicago: University of Chicago Press.

Desjarlais, Robert, and Jason Throop. 2011. "Phenomenological Approaches in Anthropology." *Annual Review of Anthropology* 40:87–102.

Dole, Christopher. 2012. *Healing Secular Life: Loss and Devotion in Modern Turkey*. Philadelphia: University of Pennsylvania Press.

Douglas, Mary. 1970. *Natural Symbols: Explorations in Cosmology*. London: Barrie & Rockliff.

Edelman, Marc. 2001. "Social Movements: Changing Paradigms and Forms of Politics." *Annual Review of Anthropology* 30:285–317.

Elinoff, Eli. 2014. "Like Everyone Else." Cultural Anthropology Online. https://culanth.org /fieldsights/572-like-everyone-else.

Ellis, Susan J., and Katherine H. Noyes. 1978. *By the People: A History of Americans as Volunteers*. Philadelphia: Energize Books.

Fabian, Johannes. 1983. *Time and the Other: How Anthropology Makes Its Object*. New York: Columbia University Press.

Farmer, Paul. 2004. "An Anthropology of Structural Violence." *Current Anthropology* 45 (3): 305–325.

Fassin, Didier. 2008. "Beyond Good and Evil? Questioning the Anthropological Discomfort with Morals." *Anthropological Theory* 8 (4): 333–344.

Fassin, Didier. 2012a. *A Companion to Moral Anthropology*. West Sussex, UK: Wiley-Blackwell.

Fassin, Didier. 2012b. *Humanitarian Reason: A Moral History of the Present*. Berkeley: University of California Press.

Fischer, Michael M. J. 2012. "Galactic Polities, Radical Egalitarianism, and the Practice of Anthropology: Tambiah on Logical Paradoxes, Social Contradictions, and Cultural Oscillations." In *Radical Egalitarianism: Local Realities, Global Relations*, edited by F. Aulino, M. Goheen, and S. J. Tambiah, 233–258. New York: Fordham University Press.

Flanders, Christopher. 2011. *About Face: Rethinking Face for 21st Century Mission*. Eugene, OR: Pickwick.

Foucault, Michel. 1988. *Technologies of the Self*. Edited by Luther H. Martin, Huck Gutman, and Patrick H. Hutton. Amherst: University of Massachusetts Press.

Friesen, Norm. 2017. "Confessional Technologies of the Self: From Seneca to Social Media." *First Monday* 22 (6). https://journals.uic.edu/ojs/index.php/fm/article/view /6750.

Garcia, Angela. 2010. *The Pastoral Clinic: Addiction and Dispossession along the Rio Grande*. Berkeley: University of California Press.

Gawande, Atul. 2014. *Being Mortal: Medicine and What Matters in the End*. New York: Metropolitan Books.

Gibson-Graham, J. K. 2014. "Rethinking the Economy with Thick Description and Weak Theory." *Current Anthropology* 55 (S9): S147–S153.

Glassman, Jim. 2008. "The 'Sufficiency Economy' as Neoliberalism: Notes from Thailand." Paper presented at the 10th International Conference on Thai Studies, Bangkok.

Glassman, Jim. 2010. "'The Provinces Elect Governments, Bangkok Overthrows Them': Urbanity, Class and Post-Democracy in Thailand." *Urban Studies* 47 (4): 1301–1323.

Glassman, Jim. 2011. "Cracking Hegemony in Thailand: Gramsci, Bourdieu and the Dialectics of Rebellion." *Journal of Contemporary Asia* 41 (1): 25–46.

Goffman, Erving. 1955. "On Face-Work: An Analysis of Ritual Elements of Social Interaction." *Psychiatry: Journal for the Study of Interpersonal Processes* 18 (3): 213–231.

Goffman, Erving. 2005 (1967). *Interaction Ritual: Essays in Face-to-Face Behavior*. Chicago: Aldine.

Good, Byron. 1994. *Medicine, Rationality, and Experience: An Anthropological Perspective*. Cambridge: Cambridge University Press.

Good, Byron. 2010. "Theorizing the 'Subject' of Medical and Psychiatric Anthropology." In *2010 R. R. Marett Memorial Lecture*. Oxford: Exeter College, Oxford University.

Good, Byron, and Mary-Jo DelVecchio Good. 1994. "In the Subjunctive Mode: Epilepsy Narratives in Turkey." *Social Science and Medicine* 38 (6): 835–842.

Good, Byron J., and Mary-Jo DelVecchio Good. 1993. "'Learning Medicine': The Constructing of Medical Knowledge at Harvard Medical School." In *Knowledge, Power, and Practice: The Anthropology of Medicine and Everyday Life*, edited by S. Lindenbaum and M. Lock, 81–107. Berkeley: University of California Press.

Good, Mary-Jo DelVecchio. 1995. *American Medicine: The Quest for Competence*. Los Angeles: University of California Press.

Good, Mary-Jo DelVecchio, Tsuenetsu Munakata, Yasuki Kobayashi, Cheryl Mattingly, and Byron Good. 1994. "Oncology and Narrative Time." *Social Science and Medicine* 38 (6): 855–862.

Goode, William J. 1978. *The Celebration of Heroes: Prestige as a Control System*. Berkeley: University of California Press.

Graeber, David. 2007. *Possibilities: Essays on Hierarchy, Rebellion, and Desire*. Oakland, CA: AK Press.

Gray, Christine. 1986. "Thailand: The Soteriological State in the 1970s." PhD Thesis, University of Chicago.

Gray, Christine. 1991. "Hegemonic Images: Language and Silence in the Royal Thai Polity." *Man* 26 (1): 43–65.

Gray, Christine. 2016. "Soul of a Nation." *New Mandala*, November 18. https://www.newmandala.org/soul-of-a-nation/.

Greenberg, Jessica, and Andrea Muehlebach. 2006. "The Old World and Its New Economy: Notes on the 'Third Age' in Western Europe Today." In *Generations and Globalization: Youth, Age, and Family in the New World Economy*, edited by J. Cole and D. Durham, 190–214. Bloomington: Indiana University Press.

Gullette, Margaret. 2004. *Aged By Culture*. Chicago: University of Chicago Press.

Hallisey, Charles, trans. 2015. *Therigatha: Poems of the first Buddhist Women*. Cambridge, MA: Harvard University Press.

Hallisey, Charles, and Hammalawa Saddhatissa. 1997. *Buddhist Ethics*. Boston: Wisdom Publications.

Hamilton, Annette. 1991. "Rumors, Foul Calumnies and the Safety of the State: Mass Media and National Identity in Thailand." In *National Identity and its Defenders: Thailand, 1939–1989*, edited by C. Reynolds, 341–379. Chiang Mai: Silkworm Books.

Han, Clara. 2012. *Life in Debt: Times of Care and Violence in Neoliberal Chile*. Berkeley: University of California Press.

Handelman, Don. 2005. "Introduction: Why Ritual in Its Own Right? How So?" In *Ritual in Its Own Right*, edited by D. Handelman and G. Lindquist, 1–32. New York: Berghahn Books.

Handler, Richard. 1986. "Authenticity." *Anthropology Today* 2 (1): 2–4.

Harris, Joseph. 2014a. "'Developmental Capture' of the State: Explaining Thailand's Universal Coverage Policy." *Journal of Health Politics, Policy and Law* 40 (1): 165–193.

Harris, Joseph. 2014b. "Who Governs? Autonomous Political Networks as a Challenge to Power in Thailand." *Journal of Contemporary Asia* 45 (1): 3–25.

Hashimoto, Akiko, and John W. Traphagan. 2008. "Changing Japanese Families." In *Imagined Families, Lived Families: Culture and Kinship in Contemporary Japan*, edited by A. Hashimoto and J. W. Traphagan, 1–12. New York: State University of New York Press.

Heim, Maria. 2011. "Buddhist Ethics: A Review Essay." *Journal of Religious Ethics* 39 (3): 571–584.

Heim, Maria. 2014. *The Forerunner of All Things: Buddhaghosa on Mind, Intention, and Agency*. Oxford: Oxford University Press.

Heim, Maria. 2017. "Buddhaghosa on the Phenomenology of Love and Compassion." In *The Oxford Handbook of Indian Philosophy*, edited by Jonardon Ganeri, 171–189. Oxford: Oxford University Press.

Heine-Geldern, Robert. 1956. "Conceptions of State and Kingship in Southeast Asia." Southeast Asia Program, Department of Far Eastern Studies, Cornell University: Data Paper Number 18.

Hendriks, Ruud. 2012. "Tackling Indifference: Clowning, Dementia, and the Articulation of a Sensitive Body." *Medical Anthropology* 31 (6): 459–476.

Herzfeld, Michael. 2002. "The Absent Presence: Discourses of Crypto-Colonialism." *South Atlantic Quarterly* 101 (4): 899–926.

Herzfeld, Michael. 2003. *The Body Impolitic: Artisans and Artifice in the Global Hierarchy of Value*. Chicago: University of Chicago Press.

Herzfeld, Michael. 2005. *Cultural Intimacy: Social Poetics in the Nation-State*. 2nd ed. New York: Routledge.

Herzfeld, Michael. 2016. *Siege of Spirits: Community and Polity in Bangkok*. Chicago: University of Chicago Press.

Hirsch, Philip. 1991. *Development Dilemmas in Rural Thailand*. Oxford: Oxford University Press.

hooks, bell. 2002. *Communion: The Female Search for Love*. New York: William Morrow.

Hu, Hsien Chin. 1944. "The Chinese Concept of Face." *American Anthropologist* 46 (1): 45–64.

Husserl, Edmund. 1970. D. Carr, trans. *The Crisis of European Sciences and Transcendental Phenomenology: An Introduction to Phenomenological Philosophy*. Evanston, IL: Northwestern University Press.

Ito, Tomomi. 2012. *Modern Thai Buddhism and Buddhadasa Bhikkhu: A Social History*. Singapore: NUS Press.

Jackson, Peter. 1989. *Buddhism, Legitimation, and Conflict: The Political Functions of Urban Thai Buddhism*. Singapore: Institute of Southeast Asian Studies.

Jackson, Peter. 2004. "The Performative State: Semi-Coloniality and the Tyranny of Images in Modern Thailand." *Sojourn* 19 (2): 219–253.

Jackson, Peter. 2016. *First Queer Voices from Thailand*. Hong Kong: Hong Kong University Press.

Jordt, Ingrid. 2007. *Burma's Mass Lay Meditation Movement*. Athens: Ohio University Press.

Juree Vichit-Vadakan. 2002. *An Overview of Philanthropy and Civil Society in Thailand*. Bangkok: Center for Philanthropy and Civil Society, National Institute of Development Administration.

Kadir, Nazima. 2016. *The Autonomous Life: Paradoxes of Hierarchy and Authority in the Squatters Movement in Amsterdam*. Manchester, UK: Manchester University Press.

Kasian Tejapira. 2015. "'Governance' in Thailand." In *A Sarong for Clio: Essays on the Intellectual and Cultural History of Thailand*, edited by M. Peleggi, 181–196. Ithaca, NY: Southeast Asia Program Publications.

Keane, Webb. 2002. "Sincerity, 'Modernity,' and the Protestants." *Cultural Anthropology* 17 (1): 65–92.

Kemp, Jeremy. 1988. *Seductive Mirage: The Search for Village Community in Southeast Asia*. Comparative Asian Studies 3. Dordrecht: Foris Publication.

Keyes, Charles. 1983. "Merit-Transference in the Karmic Theory of Popular Theravada Buddhism." In *Karma: An Anthropological Inquiry*, edited by C. Keyes and E. V. Daniel, 261–286. Berkeley: University of California Press.

Klein, Naomi. 2007. *The Shock Doctrine: The Rise of Disaster Capitalism.* New York: Picador.

Kleinman, Arthur. 2006. *What Really Matters.* Oxford: Oxford University Press.

Kleinman, Arthur. 2007. "Today's Biomedicine and Caregiving: Are They Incompatible to the Point of Divorce?" Cleveringa Lecture delivered November 26, 2007, Leiden University.

Kleinman, Arthur. 2008. "Catastrophe and Caregiving: The Failure of Medicine as an Art." *The Lancet* 371:22–23.

Kleinman, Arthur. 2009. "Caregiving: The Odyssey of Becoming More Human." *The Lancet* 373:192–193.

Kleinman, Arthur. 2011. "The Divided Self, Hidden Values, and Moral Sensibility in Medicine." *The Lancet* 377 (March 5): 804–805.

Kleinman, Arthur, and Joan Kleinman. 1993. "Face, Favor and Families: The Social Course of Mental Health Problems in Chinese and American Societies." *Chinese Journal of Mental Health* 6:37–47.

Klima, Alan. 2002. *The Funeral Casino: Meditation, Massacre, and Exchange with the Dead in Thailand.* Princeton, NJ: Princeton University Press.

Knodel, John, and Napaporn Chayovan. 2009. "Older Persons in Thailand: A Demographic, Social and Economic Profile." *Ageing International* 33:3–14.

Knodel, John, Vipan Prachuabmoh, and Napaporn Chayovan. 2013. *The Changing Well-Being of the Thai Elderly: An Update from the 2011 Survey of Older Persons in Thailand.* Vol. 13–793. Ann Arbor, MI: Population Studies Center.

Knodel, John, and Bussarawan Teerawichitchainan. 2017. "Family Support for Older Persons in Thailand: Challenges and Opportunities." University of Michigan Population Studies Center Research Report 17-879. Ann Arbor: University of Michigan.

Kohn, Eduardo. 2013. *How Forests Think: Toward an Anthropology beyond the Human.* Berkeley: University of California Press.

Laderman, Carol, and Marina Roseman. 1996. *The Performance of Healing.* New York: Routledge.

Laidlaw, James. 2002. "For an Anthropology of Ethics and Freedom." *Journal of the Royal Anthropological Institute* 8:311–332.

Lamb, Sarah. 2009. "Elder Residences and Outsourced Sons: Remaking Aging in Cosmopolitan India." In *The Cultural Context of Aging,* edited by J. Sokolovsky, 418–440. Westport, CT: Praeger.

Lamb, Sarah. 2014. "Permanent Personhood or Meaningful Decline? Toward a Critical Anthropology of Successful Aging." *Journal of Aging Studies* 29:41–52.

Lambek, Michael. 2010. *Ordinary Ethics: Anthropology, Language, and Action.* New York: Fordham University Press.

Leach, Edmund. 1954. *Political Systems of Highland Burma: A Study of Kachin Social Structure.* London: Athlone Press.

Lichter, David, and Laurence Epstein. 1983. "Irony in Tibetan Notions of the Good Life." In *Karma: An Anthropological Inquiry,* edited by C. Keyes and E. V. Daniel, 223–260. Berkeley: University of California Press.

Livingston, Julie. 2012. *Improvising Medicine: An African Oncology Ward in an Emerging Cancer Epidemic.* Durham, NC: Duke University Press.

Long, Susan Orpett. 2005. *Final Days: Japanese Culture and Choice at the End of Life.* Honolulu: University of Hawai'i Press.

Lopez, Donald. 2002. *Modern Buddhist Bible: Essential Readings from East and West.* Boston: Beacon Press.

Luhrmann, Tanya. 2011. "Toward an Anthropological Theory of Mind." *Suomen Antropologi: Journal of the Finnish Anthropological Society* 36 (4 Winter): 5–13.

Mahmood, Saba. 2012. "Ethics and Piety." In *A Companion to Moral Anthropology*, edited by D. Fassin, 223–239. Malden, MA: Wiley-Blackwell.

Marietta, Don E. 1970. "Conscience in Greek Stoicism." *Numen* 17(3): 176–187.

Martin, Aryn, Natasha Myers, and Ana Viseu. 2015. "The Politics of Care in Technoscience." *Social Studies of Science* 45 (5): 625–641.

Mattingly, Cheryl. 1998. *Healing Dramas and Clinical Plots: The Narrative Structure of Experience.* Cambridge: Cambridge University Press.

Mattingly, Cheryl. 2014. *Moral Laboratories: Family Peril and the Struggle for a Good Life.* Berkeley: University of California Press.

McCargo, Duncan. 2005. "Network Monarchy and Legitimacy Crises in Thailand." *Pacific Review* 18 (4): 499–519.

McCargo, Duncan, and Patthamānan Ukrist. 2005. *The Thaksinization of Thailand.* Copenhagen: NIAS Press.

McDaniel, Justin. 2008. *Gathering Leaves and Lifting Words: Histories of Buddhist Monastic Education in Laos and Thailand.* Seattle: University of Washington Press.

McDaniel, Justin. 2011. *The Lovelorn Ghost and the Magical Monk: Practicing Buddhism in Modern Thailand.* New York: Columbia University Press.

McMahan, David L. 2008. *The Making of Buddhist Modernism.* Oxford: Oxford University Press.

Merleau-Ponty, Maurice. 2004. *Maurice Merleau-Ponty: Basic Writings.* Edited by Thomas Baldwin. London: Routledge, Taylor and Francis.

Milligan, Christine, and David Conradson. 2006. *Landscapes of Voluntarism: New Spaces of Health, Welfare and Governance.* Bristol, UK: Policy Press at the University of Bristol.

Mol, Annemarie. 2008. *The Logic of Care: Health and the Problem of Patient Choice.* London: Routledge.

Mol, Annemarie, Ingunn Moser, and Jeannette Pols. 2010. *Care in Practice: On Tinkering in Clinics, Homes and Farms.* Bielefel, Netherlands: Transcript.

Montgomery, Nick, and carla bergman. 2017. *Joyful Militancy: Building Resistance in Toxic Times.* Chico, CA: AK Press.

Morris, Rosalind. 1995. "All Made Up: Performance Theory and the New Anthropology of Sex and Gender." *Annual Review of Anthropology* 24:567–592.

Morris, Rosalind. 2002. "Crises of the Modern in Northern Thailand: Ritual, Tradition, and the New Value of Pastness." In *Cultural Crisis and Social Memory: Modernity and Identity in Thailand and Laos*, edited by S. Tanabe and C. F. Keyes, 68–94. New York: RoutledgeCurzon.

Muehlebach, Andrea. 2012. *The Moral Neoliberal: Welfare and Citizenship in Italy.* Chicago: University of Chicago Press.

Mulder, Niels. 2000. *Inside Thai Society: Religion, Everyday Life, Change.* Chiang Mai: Silkworm Books.

Murphy, Michelle. 2015. "Unsettling Care: Troubling Transnational Itineraries of Care in Feminist Health Practices." *Social Studies of Science* 45 (5): 717–737.

NCE (National Commission of the Elderly). 2004. *Situation of the Thai Elderly.* Bangkok: Bureau of Empowerment for Older Persons, Thai Ministry of Social Development and Human Security.

Needham, Rodney. 1972. *Belief, Language, and Experience.* Chicago: University of Chicago Press.

Nguyen, Vinh-Kim. 2010. *The Republic of Therapy: Triage and Sovereignty in West Africa's Time of AIDS.* Durham, NC: Duke University Press.

Pasuk Phongpaichit and Chris Baker. 1996. *Thailand's Boom.* Chiang Mai: Silkworm Books.

Pasuk Phongpaichit and Chris Baker. 2000. *Thailand's Crisis.* Chiang Mai: Silkworm Books.

Pasuk Phongpaichit and Chris Baker. 2002. *Pluto-Populism in Thailand: Business Remaking Politics*. pioneer.chula.ac.th/~ppasuk/plutopopulism.pdf.

Pasuk Phongpaichit and Chris Baker. 2004. *Thaksin: The Business of Politics in Thailand*. Chiang Mai: Silkworm Books.

Payutto, P. A. 1995. *Buddhist Solutions for the 21st Century*. B. Evans, transl. Bangkok: Buddhadhamma Foundation.

Payutto, P. A. 2001. *Thai Buddhism in the Buddhist World*. Bangkok: Buddhadhamma Foundation.

Persons, Larry Scott. 2008a. "The Anatomy of Thai Face." *Manusya: Journal of Humanities* 11 (1): 53–75.

Persons, Larry Scott. 2008b. *Face Dynamics, Social Power and Virtue among Thai Leaders: A Cultural Analysis*. PhD Thesis, Fuller Theological Seminary, Pasadena, CA.

Phillips, Herbert P. 1965. *Thai Peasant Personality: The Patterning of Interpersonal Behavior in the Village of Bang Chan*. Berkeley: University of California Press.

Pongsapich, Amara. 1995. "Nongovernmental Organizations in Thailand." In *Emerging Civil Societies in the Asia Pacific Community*, edited by T. Yamamoto, 245–270. Singapore: Institute of Southeast Asian Studies and Japan Center for International Exchange.

Povinelli, Elizabeth. 2011. *Economies of Abandonment: Social Belonging and Endurance in Late Liberalism*. Durham, NC: Duke University Press.

Puett, Michael. 2012. "Economies of Ghosts, Gods, and Goods: The History and Anthropology of Chinese Temple Networks." In *Radical Egalitarianism: Local Realities, Global Relations*, edited by F. Aulino, M. Goheen, and S. J. Tambiah, 91–100. New York: Fordham University Press.

Puett, Michael. 2014. "Ritual Disjunctions: Ghosts, Philosophy, and Anthropology." In *The Ground Between: Anthropologists Engage Philosophy*, edited by V. Das, M. Jackson, A. Kleinman, and B. Singh, 218–233. Durham, NC: Duke University Press.

Puig de la Bellacasa, Maria. 2017. *Matters of Care: Speculative Ethics in More Than Human Worlds*. Minneapolis: University of Minnesota Press.

Putnam, Robert. 2000. *Bowling Alone: The Collapse and Revival of American Community*. New York: Simon and Schuster.

Razsa, Maple. 2015. *Bastards of Utopia: Living Radical Politics after Socialism*. Bloomington: Indiana University Press.

Reeler, Anne V. 1996. *Money and Friendship: Modes of Empowerment in Thai Health Care*. Amsterdam: Het Spinhuis.

Reynolds, Craig. 2009. "The Origins of Community in the Thai Discourse of Global Governance." In *Tai Lands and Thailand: Community and State in Southeast Asia*, edited by A. Walker, 27–43. Honolulu: University of Hawai'i Press.

Robbins, Joel. 2007. "Between Reproduction and Freedom: Morality, Value, and Radical Cultural Change." *Ethnos* 72 (3): 293–314.

Robbins, Joel. 2009. "Value, Structure, and the Range of Possibilities: A Response to Zigon." *Ethnos* 74 (2): 277–285.

Rudnyckyj, Daromir. 2011. "Circulating Tears and Managing Hearts: Governing through Affect in an Indonesian Steel Factory." *Anthropological Theory* 11 (1): 63–87.

Sawicki, Marianne. 1998. "Personal Connections: The Phenomenology of Edith Stein." In *Yearbook of the Irish Philosophical Society* (2004), 148–169. Maynooth, Ireland: Irish Philosophical Society.

Schedneck, Brooke. 2015. *Thailand's International Meditation Centers: Tourism and the Global Commodification of Religious Practices*. London: Routledge.

Scheper-Hughes, Nancy, and Margaret M. Lock. 1987. "The Mindful Body: A Prolegomenon to Future Work in Medical Anthropology." *Medical Anthropology Quarterly* 1 (1): 6–41.

Scott, James. 1998. *Seeing Like a State*. New Haven, CT: Yale University Press.

Seligman, Adam B., Robert P. Weller, Michael J. Puett, and Bennett Simon. 2008. *Ritual and Its Consequences: An Essay on the Limits of Sincerity*. Oxford: Oxford University Press.

Shohet, Merav. 2013. "Everyday Sacrifice and Language Socialization in Vietnam: The Power of a Respect Particle." *American Anthropologist* 115 (2): 203–217.

Silver, Nate. 2011. "Where to Get the World's Best Service." *New York Times Magazine*, August 7.

Simpkins, Dulcey. 2003. "Radical Influence on the Third Sector: Thai N.G.O. contributions to Socially Responsive Politics." In *Radicalising Thailand: New Political Perspectives*, edited by J. G. Ungpakorn, 253–288. Bangkok: Institute of Asian Studies, Chulalongkorn University.

Sinnott, Megan. 2004. *Toms and Dees: Transgender Identity and Female Same-Sex Relationships in Thailand*. Honolulu: University of Hawai'i Press.

Sokolovsky, Jay. 2009. *The Cultural Context of Aging: Worldwide Perspectives*. 3rd ed. Westport, CT: Praeger.

Sommai Premchit and Amphay Dore. 1992. *The Lan Na Twelve-Month Traditions*. Chiang Mai: Sommai Premchit and Amphay Dore, with support from the Toyota Foundation.

Sopranzetti, Claudio. 2013. "A Return to Regulated Neoliberalism." Conference Paper. SSRC InterAsia, Istanbul, October.

Sopranzetti, Claudio. 2018. *Owners of the Map: Motorcycle Taxi Drivers, Mobility, and Politics in Bangkok*. Berkeley: University of California Press.

Stein, Edith. 1989 (1917). *On the Problem of Empathy*. W. Stein, transl. Washington, DC: ICS Publications.

Stevenson, Lisa. 2014. *Life beside Itself: Imagining Care in the Canadian Arctic*. Berkeley: University of California Press.

Stoller, Paul. 1984. "Sound in Songhay Cultural Experience." *American Ethnologist* 11 (3): 559–570.

Stonington, Scott. 2009. *The Uses of Dying: Ethics, Politics and End of Life in Buddhist Thailand*. PhD Thesis, Department of Anthropology, University of California–San Francisco and University of California–Berkeley.

Stonington, Scott. 2011. "Facing Death, Gazing Inward: End-of-Life and the Transformation of Clinical Subjectivity in Thailand." *Culture, Medicine and Psychiatry* 35:113–133.

Stonington, Scott. 2012. "On Ethical Locations: The Good Death in Thailand, Where Ethics Sits in Places." *Social Science and Medicine* 75:836–844.

Stout, Jeffrey. 2010. *Blessed Are the Organized: Grassroots Democracy in America*. Princeton, NJ: Princeton University Press.

Streckfuss, David. 2011. *Truth on Trial in Thailand: Defamation, Treason, and Lèse-Majesté*. London: Routledge.

Stryker, Susan. 2006. "(De)Subjugated Knowledges: An Introduction to Transgender Studies." In *The Transgender Studies Reader*, edited by S. Stryker and S. Whittle, 1–18. New York: Routledge.

Suntaree Komin. 1990. *Psychology of the Thai People*. Bangkok: Research Center, National Institute of Development Administration (NIDA).

Supasawad Chardchawarn. 2008. "Decentralization under Threat? Impacts of the CEO Governor Policy upon Thai Local Government." In *Local Government in Thailand— Analysis of the Local Administrative Organization Survey*, edited by F. Nagai, N. Mektrairat, and T. Funatsu, 31–50. Institute of Developing Economies–Japan External Trade Organization. http://www.ide.go.jp/English/Publish/Download/Jrp/147.html.

Sutthichai Jitapunkul, Napaporn Chayovan, and Jiraporn Kespichayawattana. 2002. "National Policies on Ageing and Long-Term Care Provision for Older Persons in Thailand." In *Ageing and Long-Term Care: National Policies in the Asia-Pacific*, edited by D. R. Phillips and A. C. M. Chan, 181–213. Singapore: Institute of Southeast Asian Studies.

Tambiah, Stanley J. 1976. *World Conqueror and World Renouncer: A Study of Buddhism and Polity in Thailand against a Historical Background*. Cambridge: Cambridge University Press.

Tambiah, Stanley J. 1979. *A Performative Approach to Ritual: Radcliffe-Brown Lecture 1979*. Oxford: Oxford University Press.

Tanabe, Shigeharu. 1991. "Spirits, Power and the Discourse of Female Gender: The Phi Meng Cult of Northern Thailand." In *Thai Constructions of Knowledge*, edited by Manas Chitakasem and A. Turton, 183–212. London: School of Oriental and African Studies, University of London.

Tausig, Benjamin. 2013. *Bangkok Is Ringing*. New York: New York University.

Taylor, Janelle. 2008. "On Recognition, Caring, and Dementia." *Medical Anthropology Quarterly* 22 (4): 313–335.

Taylor, Marilyn. 2002. "Government, the Third Sector and the Contract Culture: The UK Experience So Far." In *Dilemmas of the Welfare Mix: The New Structure of Welfare in an Era of Privatization*, edited by Ugo Ascoli and Costanzo Ranci, 77–108. New York: Kluwer Academic/Plenum.

Temsak Phungrassami, Hutcha Sriplung, Aran Roka, Em-nasree Mintrasak, Thanarpan Peerawong, and Umard Aegem. 2003. "Disclosure of a Cancer Diagnosis in Thai Patients Treated with Radiotherapy." *Social Science and Medicine* 57:1675–1682.

Thaworn Sakunphanit and Worawet Suwanrada. 2011. "500 Baht Universal Pension Scheme." In *Sharing Innovative Experiences: Successful Social Protection Floor Experiences*. Vol. 18. Edited by I. S. S. U.-N. Experts, 401–415. New York: Global South-South Development Academy, United National Development Programme.

Thongchai Winichakul. 1994. *Siam Mapped: A History of the Geo-Body of a Nation*. Honolulu: University of Hawai'i Press.

Throop, Jason. 2008. "On the Problem of Empathy: The Case of Yap, Federated States of Micronesia." *Ethos* 36 (4): 402–426.

Throop, Jason, and Keith M. Murphy. 2002. "Bourdieu and Phenomenology: A Critical Assessment." *Anthropological Theory* 2 (2): 185–207.

Ticktin, Miriam. 2011. *Casualties of Care: Immigration and the Politics of Humanitarianism in France*. Berkeley: University of California Press.

Ting-Toomey, Stella. 1994. "Face and Facework: An Introduction." In *The Challenge of Facework: Cross-Cultural Interpersonal Issues*, edited by S. Ting-Toomey, 1–14. Albany: State University of New York Press.

Traphagan, John W. 2004. *The Practice of Concern: Ritual, Well-Being, and Aging in Rural Japan*. Durham, NC: Carolina Academic Press.

Trilling, Lionel. 1972. *Sincerity and Authenticity*. Cambridge, MA: Harvard University Press.

Tronto, Joan C. 1993. *Moral Boundaries: A Political Argument for an Ethic of Care*. New York: Routledge.

Ukosakul, Margaret. 2003. "Conceptual Metaphors Motivating the Use of Thai 'Face.'" In *Cognitive Linguistics and Non-Indo-European Languages*, edited by E. H. Casad and G. B. Palmer, 275–304. Berlin: Mouton de Gruyter.

Vandergeest, Peter. 1996. "Real Villages: National Narratives of Rural Development." In *Creating the Countryside: The Politics of Rural and Environmental Discourse*, edited by E. M. Dupuis and P. Vandergeest, 279–302. Philadelphia: Temple University Press.

Van Esterik, Penny. 2000. *Materializing Thailand*. Oxford: Berg.

Varela, Francisco J. 1999. *Ethical Know-How: Action, Wisdom, and Cognition*. Stanford, CA: Stanford University Press.

Varela, Francisco J., Eleanor Rosch, and Evan Thompson. 1992. *The Embodied Mind: Cognitive Science and Human Experience*. Cambridge, MA: MIT Press.

Wheeler, Matt. 2010. "People's Patron or Patronizing the People? The Southern Border Provinces Administrative Centre in Perspective." *Contemporary Southeast Asia* 32 (2): 208–233.

Wijeyewardene, Gehan. 1986. *Place and Emotion in Northern Thai Ritual Behavior*. Bangkok: Pandora.

williams, Rev. angel Kyodo, Lama Rod Owens, and Jashime Syedullah. 2016. *Radical Dharma: Talking Race, Love, and Liberation*. Berkeley, CA: North Atlantic Books.

Wilson, Ara. 2004. *The Intimate Economies of Bangkok: Tomboys, Tycoons and Avon Ladies in the Global City*. Berkeley: University of California Press.

Wilson, Ara. 2016. "The Infrastructure of Intimacy." *Signs: Journal of Women in Culture and Society* 41 (2): 1–34.

Yamamoto, Tadashi. 1995. *Emerging Civil Societies in the Asia Pacific Community*. Singapore/Tokyo: Institute of Southeast Asian Studies/ Japan Center for International Exchange.

Yang, Lawrence Hsin, and Arthur Kleinman. 2008. "'Face' and the Embodiment of Stigma in China: The Cases of Schizophrenia and AIDS." *Social Science and Medicine* 67 (3): 398–408.

Zelizer, Viviana. 2010. "Caring Everywhere." In *Intimate Labors: Cultures, Technologies, and the Politics of Care*, edited by E. Boris and R. S. Parreñas, 267–279. Stanford, CA: Stanford University Press.

Zigon, Jarrett. 2008. *Morality: An Anthropological Perspective*. Oxford: Berg.

Zigon, Jarrett. 2009a. "Phenomenological Anthropology and Morality: A Reply to Robbins." *Ethnos* 74 (2): 286–288.

Zigon, Jarrett. 2009b. "Within a Range of Possibilities: Morality and Ethics in Social Life." *Ethnos* 74 (2): 251–276.

โกมาตร จึงเสถียรทรัพย์ [Komatra Cheungsatiansup] et al. 2550 (2007). อาสาสมัครสาธารณสุข จิตอาสา กับสุขภาวะไทย [Public Health Volunteers: The Spirit of Volunteering and Health in Thailand]. Nonthaburi: สำนักวิจัยสังคมและสุขภาพ (สวสส.) [Society and Health Institute (SHI)].

คณะรัฐมนตรีชุดพลเอก สุรยุทธ์ จุลานนท์ (นายกรัฐมนตรี) [The Cabinet of General Surayud Chulanont (Prime Minister)]. 2550 (2007). นโยบายด้านการคุ้มครองสถานภาพผู้สูงอายุ โดยการขยายผลการ ดำเนินงานโครงการอาสาสมัครดูแลผู้สูงอายุที่บ้าน [Policy for Extending Volunteers for the Elderly].

คำ ผกา [Kam Pagaa]. 2553 (2010). "ไม่เถียงแต่ด่า" [Not to Argue, but Abuse]. มติชน สุดสัปดาห์ [Matichon Weekly]. 3–9 ก.ย. [September].

จารุประภา วะสี และ มัณฑนา บรรณาธรรม [Jaarubprapaa Wasii and Mantanaa Banaatam]. เรื่องเล่าจิตอาสา [Tales of Spirit Volunteers]. Bangkok: ศูนย์ส่งเสริมและพัฒนาพลังแผ่นดินเชิง คุณธรรม [Center for Moral Ethics] and สำนักงานบริหารและพัฒนาองค์ความรู้ [Office of Management and Development of Knowledge].

ลือชัย ศรีเงินยวง และ ยงยุทร พงษ์สุภาธ [Leuchai Sringernyuang and Yongyut Ponsupap]. 2009. Primary Care vs. Primary Health Care: พัฒนาการและข้อเสนอทศวรรษที่สี่การสาธารณสุขมูลฐาน ไทย [Primary Care vs. Primary Health Care: Development and Recommendations]. Nonthoburi, Thailand: สถาบันวิจัยระบบสาธารณสุข (สวรส.) [Health Systems Research Institute (HSRI)].

นพ นันทวัน [Nop Nantwan]. 2548 (2005). เจ้ากรรมจองเวร [*Chaokam Chŏngwēn*, Karmic Retribution]. Bangkok: ไพลิน [Palin Publishers].

พระไพศาล วิสาโล and ปรีดา เรืองวิชาธร [Pra Paisal Wisalo and Bprida Reungwichatawn]. 2549 (2006). เผชิญความตายอย่างสงบ: สาระและกระบวนการเรียนรู้ [Approaching Death Peacefully: Meaning and Process]. Bangkok: เครือข่ายพุทธิกา [Phuthikā Network].

ราช รามัญ [Rat Raman]. 2551 (2008). DNA กรรม [Karma DNA]. Bangkok: ไพลินบุ๊คเน็ต [Palin Booknet].

สถาบันไทยรูรัลเนท [Thai Rural Net]. 2550 (2007). กฎหมายที่เกี่ยวข้องกับ อาสาสมัครและการให้ [Laws Concerning Volunteers and Giving]. volunteerspirit.org.

สนิท สมัครการ [Sanit Samarkangaan]. 2518 (1975). เรื่อง "หน้า" ของคนไทย วิเคราะห์ตามแนวคิดทาง มานุษยวิทยาภาษาศาสตร์ [Concerning the "Face" of Thai People: Analysis According to the Linguistic Anthropology Approach]. *Thai Journal of Development Administration* 15 (4): 492–505.

สุธาทิพย์ แก้วเกลี้ง [Sutaatip Gaewgaliyang]. 2549 (2006). การพัฒนาจิตอาสา แนวพุทธศาสนา [The Development of Buddhist Volunteer Spirit]. Bangkok: Mahidol University, Department of Religious Studies.

Index

Abhidhammic theory of mind, 14–15, 44, 48–53; agency and, 147–48; care and, 15–16; Christianity and, 66; conditioning and, 49; diagnosis shielding and, 55, 57–58, 62; emotions and, 44–45, 57–58; empathy and, 159n9, 171–72n23; equanimity and, 21, 44–45, 58; face and, 83; fields and, 72; importance of, 44–45, 50–51, 53; intentionality and, 15–16, 44–45, 49–50, 159–60n14; interdependence and, 135; karma and, 44–45, 49, 50–51, 55, 58, 66, 159n14; logic of "don't ask, don't tell" and, 45–56, 59; mental components in, 49, 55, 66; morality and, 16; restraint and, 67; self-reflection and, 66, 147–48; the social body and, 72; social change and, 18; terminology of, 154n32; volunteering and, 92, 95. *See also* Pali canon; theory of mind

Abhisit Vejjajiva, 11, 110, 139

abortion, 119, 122, 170n8

agency, 13–16, 17–18, 67, 120–26, 147–48, 153 n23, 155 n35, 163 n13, 170 n4. *See also* structural violence

aging, 3, 6–7, 11, 70, 155n6; aging society, 87, 89, 90, 93, 104, 151n6, 155n2; aging policy 6, 11, 135, 151nn3–4, 152nn17–18, 166n12, 168n25; eldercare movements in Thailand, 1–3, 6–8, 11, 56, 155n2, 151nn3–4, 151n6

Aom (Yāi Maw's eldest daughter), 19–20, 21–24, 34–36, 39–40, 88, 113, 134, 147

Aristotle, 44, 154n31, 164n30, 173n3

Asad, Talal, 24, 157n20

Asian financial crisis (1997), 9

Austin, J. L., 30

Aw Paw Saw (Volunteers Caring for Older People at Home), 11, 93–96, 98, 152n19, 167n17

Aw Saw Maw (Ministry of Public Health's volunteer program), 90, 93, 94, 99, 133–34, 152n19, 166n13, 167n17

Bell, Catherine, 35

Bellah, Robert, 22

bergman, carla, 146

Bhumibol (King), 112, 139, 140

Biehl, João, 23

Bilmes, Leela, 47, 79, 81

BKK Pundit (blog), 173n39

Bodhiraksa, 125

Boni, Stephano, 17, 155n36

Boonyuang (Yāi Maw's daughter), 1–5, 117–19, 151n2, 170n3

Botswana, caregiving in, 22–23, 156n9

Bourdieu, Pierre, 72, 75–76

Bourgois, Philippe, 114–15

Bowie, Katherine, 134, 170n10

bowing, 77, 78–79

Brahinsky, Josh, 18

Bree (head of government elder programs in Chiang Mai), 94–97, 166n12, 167n17

brown, adrienne maree, 146, 174n8

Buch, Elana, 155n6

Buddhadasa Bhikku, 124–26

Buddhaghosa, 14, 44–45, 49, 87, 117, 144, 154n31, 159n7

Buddhism: authenticity and, 38; Christianity and, 66; contemplation and, 66; cosmopolitan interpretations of, 37, 124, 157nn24–25, 159n8, 171nn11–12; dharma and, 39, 111; diagnosis shielding and, 62; elitism and, 125–26; emotions and, 53; empathy and, 130; Engaged Buddhist movement in, 5, 124, 144; face and, 83; Four Noble Truths, 171n19; idiot compassion and, 171n20; impermanence and, 130; inner orientations and, 45–46; intentionality and, 56; literalism and metaphorism in, 124–125; modern interpretations of and in, 37, 55, 124, 144, 157nn23–25, 160n22, 163n10, 169n38, 173n1; morality and, 67, 77; Noble Eightfold Path in, 50; ontological claims and, 38, 83, 116, 132, 147, 173n6; phenomenology and, 87; pity and, 129–30, 132; prevalence of, 37; "radical dharma" 146; "real Buddhism" and, 38, 103, 148; realms of beings in, 111; restraint and, 117; ritual and, 37, 38, 103; sages in, 67; samsara and, 123; science and, 103, 163n12; soteriology in, 50, 53, 65; sublime states in, 171n16; Tsu Chi model in, 167n19; variation in, 37, 162n37; violence and, 37–38, 144; volunteering and, 111. *See also* Abhidhammic theory of mind; Pali canon

Burke, Peter, 157n19

187

CPSIA information can be obtained
at www.ICGtesting.com
Printed in the USA
LVHW091754160819
627946LV00009B/67/P